# YOGA:
# THE ESSENCE OF LIFE

Alix Johnson is a Sydney-based journalist and yoga teacher. She contributes to major newspapers and magazines articles about the body, wellness and health. Since attending her first yoga class ten years ago she has been a devoted practitioner of Hatha yoga.

# YOGA:
# THE ESSENCE OF LIFE

## EIGHT YOGIS SHARE THEIR JOURNEYS

ALIX JOHNSON

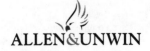

ALLEN&UNWIN

The verse on p. xviii is from *The Upanishads*, translated by Eknath
Easwaran, founder of the Blue Mountain Center of Meditation, copyright
1987; reprinted by permission of Nilgiri Press, P.O. Box 256, Tomales,
Ca 94971, *www.nilgiri.org*

First published in 2004

Allen & Unwin
83 Alexander Street
Crows Nest NSW 2065
Australia
Phone:    (61 2) 8425 0100
Fax:      (61 2) 9906 2218
Email:    info@allenandunwin.com
Web:      www.allenandunwin.com

National Library of Australia
Cataloguing-in-Publication entry:

Johnson, Alix.
   Yoga : the essence of life : eight yogis share their
   journeys.

   Bibliography.
   ISBN 1 74114 295 4.

   1. Yogis - Interviews. 2. Yoga. I. Title.

181.45

Set in 12/15 pt Dante by Bookhouse, Sydney
Printed in Australia by McPherson's Printing Group

10 9 8 7 6 5 4 3 2 1

*Our bodies are simply little whirlpools in the ocean of matter.*

Swami Vivekananda

# CONTENTS

Donna Farhi on how a holistic practice is designed to
enliven the parts of ourselves that we have shut down
to life's energy. Donna Farhi is a best-selling author of
three books on yoga. Her most recent is *Bringing Yoga to
Life: The Everyday Practice of Enlightened Living.*

Eileen Hall on striking the balance of living in the material
world while leading a spiritual life. Eileen Hall is one of
the few people in the world to be accredited to teach
yoga by Sri K. Pattabhi Jois and B.K.S. Iyengar. She is the
director of Ashtanga Yoga Moves in Sydney.

# Contents

# Contents

# PREFACE

Often what we are searching for is right before our eyes but, unaware, we go out looking for it anyway. For me, trying to find a yoga teacher who could teach me how to use the practice to better handle life was like that.

The search began on my first visit to India. I met a man in New Delhi who so closely resembled the image of the great yoga teacher B.K.S. Iyengar emblazoned on the cover of *Light on Yoga* weighing down my backpack that I instantly liked him. Invited to stroll around Connaught Place I willingly agreed and promptly followed him straight into a deserted railway yard. 'Trust me,' he purred, 'don't buy into fear.' When he suggested we 'meditate' in the quiet of an empty carriage I turned on my heels and ran. (Other than in looks, he was not related to the great yoga master from Pune.)

From Calcutta, across the northern plains, to Varanasi, through the foothills of the Himalayas and all around Rajasthan,

I searched high and low for this yoga teacher who was going to change my life. I got the idea from a book, *Yoga and Health*, that a friend had lent to me years earlier in Australia. Fate led me to my first yoga class, but it was this book that kept me there.

The book told the story of an Indian boy, Selvarajan Yesudian, who was born so sickly and weak that by the time he turned fifteen he was barely alive. Instead of standing proudly on the threshold of manhood he was mustering strength to overcome bouts of typhus, cholera and scarlet fever. His father was a famous physician to whom the wealthy of Madras flocked, but despite his vast medical knowledge he could do nothing to build the vigour of his own son.

Selvarajan tried every means available to him to become well, including yoga. Instead of curing him, one night of zealous *asana* (physical postures) and *pranayama* (rhythmic breathing exercises) left him more wasted than ever. He nearly gave up but felt pulled by an instinct for yoga to run away from his parents' home and live with the yogis in the folkloric hermitages beyond the city bounds.

Two months passed and no one had heard from him or seen him. Then one day a strapping young man walked into Selvarajan's parents' home. This man's arms and legs were muscular and lean, his chest broad and his carriage upright and graceful. This was indeed Selvarajan. The formerly sick boy grew up to become a graceful yogi, and the author of the book I was reading. His transformation held me fixed.

The book's pages were peppered with his Adonis-like photos, the chapters effusive with gratitude for his teacher and humility for the yoga that he claimed transformed him at a level far deeper than appearance. I loved the idea that practising yoga held the potential for such change, though what made a deeper impression still was the idea of these masters in India who held the power to unravel it. And so my search began.

On my second trip to India I was a little more prepared. I arrived armed with directions to the Ashtanga Yoga Research Institute in Mysore, where I would meet Sri K. Pattabhi Jois, the original teacher of this dynamic form of Hatha yoga. Although not a student of this style of yoga (there was a long wait to visit B.K.S. Iyengar's Institute in Pune) it was a starting point for trying to understand how yoga can be transformative. Tape recorder and notepad in hand I 'interviewed' the famous octogenarian, though unfortunately I didn't understand a word he said. '*Samskara?* Garlic, did you say?' I felt lost. (*Samskaras* are the subliminal impressions within our personality, accumulated over lifetimes, that form our tendencies. Pattabhi Jois likens the residual nature of *samskaras* to the smell of garlic that lingers long after the cooking is finished.)

I quizzed his students, too, about why they had forfeited the fresh fruit juice and the clean surf beaches back home in California to live temporarily with bucket showers, power failures and four a.m. wakeup calls for *asana* practice. Over cups of spiced tea they willingly explained but again I missed the message. '*Yama? Niyama?* Er, what pose is that?' (*Yamas* and *niyamas* are behavioural codes and self-disciplines that constitute an essential part of a yoga practice.)

My understanding of yoga didn't extend beyond bending and breathing on a mat and feeling fantastic afterwards. It was too rudimentary to receive what anyone was trying to pass my way. I conceded that my chances of meeting a spiritual teacher *and* being able to understand their message were nil and, despondent, I abandoned the search and booked a holiday to the Bahamas instead. There, at the Sivananda Yoga Ashram on the island of Nassau, I enjoyed practising *asana* on a timber deck overlooking crystal blue water and fine white sand. Then, unexpectedly, the resident American swamis invited me to stay. I baulked. How could I learn anything from people who lived under palm fronds down the beach from a pink Donald Trump hotel, ate Baskin-Robbins ice-cream, and who looked and sounded altogether too normal, too like me? I was looking for all the wrong signs. The opportunity was placed before me but I was too blinded by preconceptions to see.

I returned home to Sydney, resumed my usual life as a journalist and attended yoga classes when I could. Three years passed. Almost forgetting my quest altogether, it was soon to be fulfilled.

A five-week trip north turned into a year submerged in yoga in Byron Bay, in northern New South Wales, where I was exposed to a wide range of truly wonderful teachers. These men and women guided students, like myself, into the depths of the practices, deftly showing how the mat becomes a mirror that reflects the workings of the mind. They explained the belief system that underpins the practices and that, at times, acts like a life-raft when a student is feeling 'out at sea'. While the daily practice of *asana*, *pranayama* and meditation were deeply rewarding, and the study of the texts thought-provoking and inspiring, it was the life stories of these teachers that enabled me to grasp yoga as a means to understand the essence of life.

My gratitude at discovering such teachers was matched, paradoxically, by widespread frustration within the yoga community at yoga's portrayal as merely a means to relax and stretch. The more popular it became, it seemed, the less people understood its true purpose. Certainly had I not encountered these teachers, I might have missed the message too.

This then is the purpose of this book: to share stories of senior, accomplished and long-time practitioners as a way of introducing the spiritual dimension of yoga to those who are not yet familiar with it, and to remind those who are. More than that, it is a book to inspire us to live purposeful, meaningful lives.

Only three of the eight—Iyengar teacher, Glenn Ceresoli, psychologist and Satyananda trained swami, Muktanand Meannjin, and Tantric yoga teacher, Rose Baudin—were my teachers that year in Byron Bay. Others, like Shandor Remete, who developed *Chaya Samyukta*, I had heard about through the yoga grapevine; while Hatha yoga teacher, Donna Farhi, and Aghori and Ayurvedic physician, Robert E. Svoboda, I first encountered within the covers of their many and insightful books on yoga. Others still—Simon Borg Oliver, who practises Synergy-style yoga, and Eileen Hall, who teaches *ashtanga*— I have had the privilege of studying with back home in Sydney within the context of 'ordinary' life.

Typically, I met each subject only once and they each spoke about yoga as a spiritual discipline. Most spoke of lessons learnt along their path to animate the sometimes abstract concepts and philosophies of yoga. Each teacher was gracious in their willingness to talk about their life in a way that might shed light on the integrity of the practice of yoga. As a result I have not really 'written' this book so much as acted like a vessel for other people's stories that introduce or reaffirm the richness of the tradition.

I learnt a great deal about yoga and about myself in the process of researching and collecting these stories. One lesson that will perhaps be universal is that there are authentic spiritual teachers in our midst. I never had to leave for India all those years ago to find the teacher who could help me understand myself better. They were living in my world all along. And this parallels one of the ultimate lessons of yoga: the very teacher we are searching for is within.

In the words of Swami Vivekananda, who was one of the first Indians to bring yoga to the west in the late nineteenth century: 'You are the greatest book that ever was or ever will be, the infinite depository of all that is. Until the inner teacher opens, all outside teaching is in vain. It must lead to the opening of the book of the heart to have any value.'

# A BRIEF INTRODUCTION
# TO THE PRACTICE AND
# PHILOSOPHY OF YOGA

'We are all walking the same path, just carrying different backpacks.' This is how a vegetable farmer in western New South Wales explains the many and varied ways that people forge a spiritual life. For her, it is tending the land that brings her closest to God. For others, it might be congregating in a church, mosque, synagogue or temple. For a growing number of people around the world it is through yoga.

However different spiritual endeavours appear on the outside, the intention is the same: to transcend a limited individual outlook on life and to connect with an expansive God-like perspective. Buddhists refer to this as connecting with their Buddha-nature, Christians with Christ-consciousness, in yoga it is referred to as Self-realisation.

The word 'yoga', derived from the ancient language of Sanskrit, means to 'unite'. The aim of a yogi's practice is to join that which has separated. On a simple level this means unifying body and mind, on a deeper level it means perceiving the interconnectedness of the mundane and the divine, of the individual and the universal.

This challenging concept was described skilfully by Swami Vivekananda, who was one of India's great yogis. He likened the individual to a wave, the universal to the ocean. They are one and the same in essence, but separate in name and form: 'If the wave subsides, the form vanishes in a moment, and yet the form was not a delusion . . . The whole universe, therefore, is, as it were, a peculiar form; the Absolute is that ocean while you and I, and suns and stars, and everything else are various waves of that ocean . . . As soon as the wave goes, they vanish. As soon as the individual gives up this *maya*, it vanishes for him and he becomes free.' *Maya* is the illusion of an unconnected, independent existence.

If the Absolute is the 'ocean', and the individual the 'wave', then the essence of the Absolute that resides within each individual is known as the Self, the *atman*. Contemporary author and pre-eminent Vedic scholar Georg Feurstein describes the *atman* as 'the nucleus of the innermost aspect of our being'.

Realising the presence of the Self is central to all yogic philosophy, though the practices employed to reach this insight are many and varied. Just as we all cart a different 'backpack' along the spiritual path, within the yoga community itself backpacks come in many shapes and sizes. Jnana yoga is the study of sacred scriptures to know the Self. Bhakti yoga is the worship of gods and goddesses to become familiar with one's own god-nature. Karma yoga is the performance of selfless action, contributing to the world without expecting personal rewards for one's efforts. Raja yoga, also known as Patanjali's yoga, is the 'royal' yoga that follows the eightfold path. (Patanjali's

yoga encompasses Hatha yoga, the practice of physical poses.)
The overarching aim of all branches, be it Jnana yoga, Bhakti
yoga, Karma yoga or Raja yoga, is to reconnect with the Self.

This unfamiliar concept of the Self can seem confusing at
first. It does not mean to know 'oneself' better; it is not about
navel-gazing. Rather, it means to transcend the boundaries set
by name and form, likes and dislikes, age, occupation, social
status and so on, and touch the innermost part of ourselves
that contains the essence of life. This essence is said to pervade
the entirety of creation. It is explained most eloquently in the
*Katha Upanishad* (translated here by Eknath Easwaran):

> *The Self is the sun shining in the sky,*
> *The wind blowing in space; he is the fire*
> *At the altar and in the home the guest;*
> *He dwells in human beings; in gods; in truth,*
> *And in the vast firmament; he is the fish*
> *Born in water, the plant growing in the earth,*
> *The river flowing down from the mountain.*
> *For this Self is supreme!*
> (*Katha Upanishad* II.2.2)

In ancient times, as far back as 3000 BC according to modern
archaeology, the yogi intent on pursuing this path would take
their first step by renouncing the known world. In challenging
their ability to survive unsupported by familiar 'props' of name,
place and purpose they would uncover what the Self is, and
what it is not. The German writer Hermann Hesse portrayed
this scenario with exquisite clarity in his classic novel *Siddhartha*,
a fictitious account of Guatama, the Buddha's journey to
enlightenment. For a period of his journey Siddhartha lived an

ascetic life: chaste, reclusive, abstaining from the comfort of clothes and the pleasure of food.

The ancient texts record conversations between teacher and student in such a situation. The *Upanishads*, one of the key yogic texts that means literally 'to sit near', is a collection of esoteric discussions, dating as far back as 870 BC, between spiritual masters and disciples regarding the nature of life. The teacher–student relationship has always been central to the yogic tradition. Knowledge of the practices is usually passed on orally—rarely were these teachings recorded—and the transfer of understanding from guru (teacher) to *shishya* (student) is viewed as an initiation; the inheritance of information forms a lineage (*parampara*).

The *Bhagavad Gita*, 'the Song of the Lord', written around 2500 years ago, is another momentous text and one of the most beloved in Hindu nations, as it is also the fountainhead of Hindu religion. About the *Gita*, Mahatma Ghandi is famously quoted as saying: 'When doubts start to haunt me, when disappointments stare me in the face, and I see not one ray of hope on the horizon, I turn to the *Bhagavad Gita* and find a verse to comfort me; and I immediately begin to smile in the midst of overwhelming sorrow.'

The *Gita* is an episode within one of India's great epic poems, the *Maharabhata*, that relates the conversation between the warrior Prince Arjuna and his charioteer Lord Krishna that took place on the battlefield. When Arjuna realised that relatives and friends were among his enemies he was unwilling to fight on. Krishna counselled him not to back away from his duty [*dharma*]. This 'battle' is viewed as analogous to the conflict between the lower ego-mind and the Self. Inaction is not appropriate. Yoga, said Krishna, is 'awareness in action'.

A different definition is proffered in the *Yoga Sutras*, considered the most significant yoga text of all. It is a roadmap of the invisible terrain of the spiritual journey. The *Yoga Sutras* are a collection of 196 aphorisms written by the sage Patanjali around 200 BC. Mukunda Stiles, the author of a recent interpretation of *Patanjali's Yoga Sutras*, compares Patanjali's significance to yoga with the Buddha's inherent importance to Buddhism. Another popular version from the 1950s, *How to Know God* by British writer Christopher Isherwood and Swami Prabhavananda, reflects clearly and unabashedly the aim of yoga in the title.

Patanjali gives a succinct (but not conclusive) definition of yoga—*Yogah citta vrtti nirodhah* [yoga is the cessation of the fluctuations of the mind]. This does not infer that the mind will come to a complete standstill, rather 'stillness' comes when one ceases to self-identify with the tendencies of the personality. The cravings and aversions of the personality make the waters of the mind turbid. When one is able to observe desires and aversions without getting caught in their undercurrent, clarity comes and one can remain centred in the Self. Patanjali also gives a very clear blueprint on how this is to be done—this is known as the eight limbs of yoga, or *ashtanga* yoga [*ashta*, eight, *anga*, limb].

The first two limbs are: *yama* and *niyama*, the twin angels that could be called 'high thinking' and 'simple living'. Each contains a subset of five 'vows', which ensure that your behaviour, speech and thought mirror your intent.

The next two limbs are *asana* and *pranayama*, the practice of physical postures and breathing exercises respectively, which work on the physical body to make it fitter and more vital. They also work on the mental body to refine concentration and the energetic body to purify. The regular practice of *asana*

and *pranayama* can begin to reveal the tendencies of the m
towards doubt, fear, anger and other afflictive emotions,
exposing the ego or *ahamkhara* [literally, 'I-maker']. The ego
aspect of the mind is the gatekeeper between the lower mind
and the Self.

The final four limbs concern the inner practice of meditation:
*pratyahara*, turning the senses inward; *dharana*, focusing the
mind one-pointedly; *dhyana*, meditation on one's point of focus,
and *samadhi*, blissful absorption in the object of focus. These
four combine to bring one wholly into the present moment,
where no memory of the past or thought of the future can
splinter one's concentration. In living only in that moment, the
now, the yogi appreciates life for just what it is and all that it
is. They cease to expect it to be something that their ego-self
craves or loathes. In this way life becomes joyous and the
practices deeply nurturing.

To know the Self, to see life from an expansive God-like
perspective, is to be free from the desires of the ego-mind, the
limitations of the separate self and the suffering both of these
incur. This freedom [*moksha*] returns one to a state of interconnectedness with all beings, to the blissful awareness that
the essence within one is within all. In the words of leading
eastern scholar, Barbara Stoler Miller, author of *Yoga: Discipline
of Freedom* (an interpretation of the *Yoga Sutras*), the eventual
goal of yoga is 'finally to lay bare our true human identity'.

As such, yoga is a spiritual endeavour. It is a 'backpack' like
any other that carries us along the pathway, home to the Self.

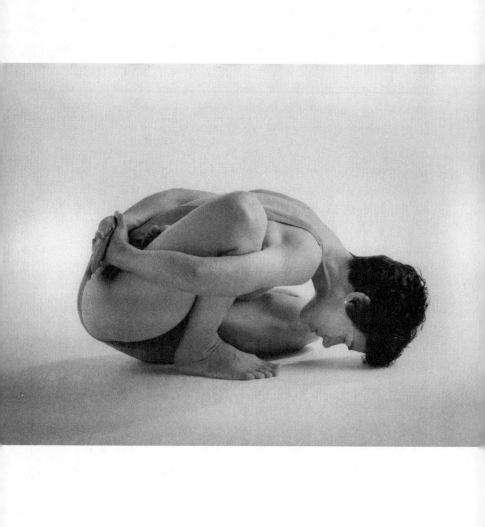

# 1

# BECOMING WHO YOU ARE

## Donna Farhi

*If you look at the sky what you tend to notice is the objects in it—the passing birds or changing clouds. The ordinary or habitual mind has a tendency to fixate and follow these transient forms without noticing the unchanging and ever present canvas of the sky. When we bring our attention to rest upon this canvas, we find that it is still, luminous, and silent. A mind filled with such awareness has become awakened to its true nature . . . We must learn to see the sky and to focus our attention on this unchanging background.*

Donna Farhi, *Yoga Mind, Body & Spirit:*
*A Return to Wholeness*

When the ten-year-old daughter of a non-practising Jew and lapsed Catholic moved from America to New Zealand she found herself uprooted from the world she knew and transplanted into a culture she did not understand. Her solution was to find her own community, to search for her own sense of belonging, and to connect deeply with a sense of self that felt more expansive than her nationality or religion could permit. This journey became a lifetime's work and the young girl is now the 44-year-old yoga teacher and author, Donna Farhi.

For nearly three decades now Donna has practised Hatha yoga and established herself as one of its leading teachers in the west. Her work is a physical exploration of what it means to be fully alive, to probe the aspects of ourselves—physical, mental, emotional, spiritual—that, for whatever reason, we have denied the breath of life. Through asana practice, the practice of physical postures, she encourages a softening of the body, mind and heart in order to eventually open the innermost doors of our being and reveal our true essence.

Donna Farhi is the author of three books on yoga: The Breathing Book; Yoga Mind, Body & Spirit: A Return to Wholeness; and Bringing Yoga to Life: The Everyday Practice of Enlightened Living. During our conversation Donna sits dappled in soft afternoon light, radiating gentleness and stillness. Her body is petite and compact, her legs curled up on the sofa and her eyes dark and perceptive; luminous pearl earrings magnify her feminine energy. She speaks in a calm and measured voice about her earliest memories of yoga. She quips that if yoga can bring peace and contentment to her life, then it can do so for anyone. She explains how her approach to yoga has enabled her to reconnect with the deepest, most constant part of her being—what she calls the natural mind, that exists beyond place and before time.

# YOGA FINDS YOU

I don't think you come to yoga, I think yoga comes to you. I was sixteen and my family was in crisis. I found myself in a foreign culture and at a new high school where yoga was offered as an elective. In those days only the really weird, nerdy kids would sign up for something like yoga. About seven of us did. The other seventy students went ice-skating! After the first class, I walked home from school and I knew within myself that this was something I was going to do every day of my life. And it was.

My first teacher wasn't really a yoga teacher, but a heavily pregnant physical education instructor who had read a few books. Because she was pregnant, the course soon finished. I asked if I could go into this tiny room in the school grounds during my elective period and continue to practise yoga by myself. Well, the principal couldn't believe that a sixteen-year-old would be practising yoga alone in a windowless, concrete room. He was so convinced that I was playing truant during this hour and a half that I got called into his office. He discovered that, yes indeed, I was practising yoga by myself in this little room, and he left it at that. So that's how I started.

Even before that, though, I was a very physical child. I was constantly dancing. I remember being sent, at about the age of seven, on a holiday to the sea-side in New Zealand with an English family. I used to love being close to the ocean. I'd dance, twirl and leap as the sea rolled in and washed out. Or I'd pretend to be a horse leaping and galloping over crashing waves. I had no self-consciousness about acting like this at all. There I'd be at the beach—Isadora Duncan doing her thing!—and I remember the mother of the girl I was staying with saying to me, 'Would you please stop that! Why can't you be more like Elizabeth?' That was one of the first moments I realised that what I was doing, which up until that moment had felt very wonderful and joyous, was not accepted. I realised that it was outside of the cultural context in which I lived, and rather than shut down my impulse to move, I began to go underground, which is what most children do.

I don't know where the impulse to move came from, because my parents aren't physical at all. My father has a genius IQ, and is an electronic engineer. I'm grateful for those genes, because I think he's given me the ability to structure my thoughts. Nor is my mother a physical person; she's never done a yoga exercise in her life. I think they still believe this is a phase I'm going through! But they're respectful and very supportive of what I do, even though they've never watched me teach a class.

At about the same time I started yoga, I began studying dance. At nineteen, I moved back to the States to take on a scholarship and I was studying classical ballet and contemporary dance full-time until I was twenty-three. Throughout that whole time I was also practising yoga, although it was very much in the background.

At about the age of twenty-three, I began to feel that all my dance training had just produced a machine. I didn't feel like I had any inner impulse for movement anymore. I was a technically proficient machine and yet my original reason for dancing was that I felt most connected to God when I was moving. I'd lost that feeling and I knew I needed to find it again, whatever the measure.

I literally stopped dancing, cold turkey. I walked out of the ballet studio one day and I didn't go back. In retrospect, that was a very radical thing to do because my entire identity was bound up in being a dancer—I never thought that I would be able to stop dancing and still live. But my need to find the inner content of myself was stronger. Because my natural proclivity was to use movement as my vessel for that search, I began studying yoga formally.

Just about the first thing I did when I started to study yoga full-time was get badly injured. I went to a class where the teacher was extremely authoritarian and she perhaps misread my ability. As a dancer, I must have looked very proficient, when really I did not have a good understanding of things like headstand variations. I went into an inverted posture and felt immediately there was something wrong and so I came down. The teacher insisted that this was not my experience. She contradicted my perception of what was going on and insisted I go back up. I went back up and herniated a disc in my neck.

I studied mostly at the Iyengar Institute in San Francisco where I did the two-year full-time teacher training course. My primary teacher was Judith Lasater, who was also a physical therapist and has a PhD in east/west psychology. My other primary teacher was Dona Holleman, who was a senior Iyengar teacher at the time and has since moved into her own way of teaching. I also travelled to India, Greece and Britain to study with different senior teachers.

At about the same time, in 1982, I started to write for *Yoga Journal*. There was a wonderful editor there, Linda Cogozzo, who nurtured me as a writer. It was quite scary to write back then, because I still was within the Iyengar system, which was very pedantic, and anyone who was writing about *asana* was a dartboard: you had better have it right—whatever right was—and of course, you could never be right!

In my early years of writing, I was always worried about whether what I was saying would be accepted or criticised. It wasn't until I got to the point where I couldn't give a damn about what anybody thought that I think my writing became more truthful. You can't write the way I do, which is as I speak, and be self-conscious and worry about every other sentence and what x, y and z is going to say when they read it or which faculty member will pull you up on which point. So long as you're very worried about what other people think, you're going to modify yourself all the time in order to be acceptable to others. And yet what people are accepting isn't really *you*— it's just whatever you've projected to please them.

Meanwhile, my yoga study began to echo a familiar pattern. What I'd done in the past was choose a very technically demanding, form-orientated kind of dance that I took to the nth degree, only to arrive at the conclusion that it wasn't working. With yoga, I did exactly the same thing. I chose a form of yoga in which the focus was more on the goal than the process, more on the form than the content. It was extremely ambitious, extremely competitive and I took it to the nth degree, coming to almost exactly the same place I had reached when I stopped dancing. I had lost the inner impulse. What's calling me to do this? What is the inner content of this practice? I couldn't answer those questions anymore.

In *The Breathing Book*, to explain how this felt I use an analogy of the botanist who spends years cultivating the perfect rose. This rose no longer has thorns, it has a long stem, a perfect bloom and is the ideal colour, but it doesn't have a fragrance anymore. For me, that's how it felt both with dance and with the system of yoga I was practising. They were without essence. I became just a shell.

I would have been just on the cusp of thirty when I realised that I could not in good conscience continue practising or teaching yoga in the methods I had been taught, despite being very grateful for the theoretical background. It was a bit like learning scales—but who wants to play scales for the rest of their lives? That's what I saw in yoga: people who weren't playing music, just scales.

It is said that we have to make the same mistake a number of times until we learn the lesson. I began questioning the obsessive focus on form in the Iyengar yoga I was practising. It seemed that the posture had become more important than the person doing it and the process they went through to achieve it. Because I had always practised any form of movement in a very organic way, to practise yoga mechanically felt at odds with what I knew and felt from my own experience.

At around that time I met a teacher who opened up a door for me to follow my heart, to follow my intuitive sense and to strike out on my own, which is what I did. Back then, leaving the Iyengar system was like being cast outside the village gates and into darkness. I was led to believe that it would mean the end of my teaching career, that I probably wouldn't survive as a teacher outside the formal Iyengar system. And in the beginning it *was* very hard.

For one thing, it was hard to find students who were interested in anything but form. I think that is still true to some degree today. And, to be fair, in the beginning I was floundering in my attempts to codify a way of taking people through this process of using asana and movement as a means to connect with God, with one's inner content. At this point, my life got really tough. I thought to myself, 'It's got to be easier than this', so I planned to go back to university and see if I could find some sort of structure I could work within.

I went for an interview at an alternative university where they were doing consciousness study programs. I told the interviewer what I was doing: 'Well,' I explained, 'I'm writing articles for *Yoga Journal* and I've been teaching yoga for five years.' He paused for a long time and eventually said, 'There's nothing here for you. Our students graduate so that they can do what you're already doing.' He told me that the composer Schoenberg did his best work when he was still struggling to find some kind of structure for his music. 'You have to find where that is for yourself,' he said. Our conversation helped me understand that the work I needed to do was explorative, not prescribed, and to embrace that. I went out onto the streets of San Francisco, walked through Chinatown, and cried because, once again, the onus was back on me to find my own solution.

At about this time, when I had broken away from pretty much everything I knew and everything that was secure and stable in my life, I met my mentor. All the teachers I've mentioned have been mentors to me, but my main mentor in life was a man named Ray Worring. Ray was like a grandfather figure who, in his own way, cared for me enormously. He was a very unorthodox teacher, and he wasn't a yoga teacher, but more than anybody, he reminded me of what I am here to do and why it is important for me to do it. The best way to describe his work was to call him a world-class psychic.

We met in what can only be described as extraordinary circumstances. We lived in different states in the U.S. and during that period, when my life was extremely painful, Ray saw a picture of me in a brochure advertising a yoga retreat and realised I was in trouble. He called me across three state lines to tell me I was at a critical juncture in my life and wanted to help me. Would I fly to Montana and wo him? (He believed in 'therapy without an office'.) I said, 'I don't mean to be rude, but you don't know me from a bar of soap. Why should you care?' He didn't miss a beat; he replied, 'There are no strangers to me in this world.'

This idea is central to the meaning of yoga: we are all from the same source. If I am refusing something in myself, then I'm refusing something in you. There are no strangers in this world. At the time when Ray called me, I was financially in ruins. I said to him, 'I have no money, I can't pay you', and he said, 'It doesn't matter, come.'

Ray literally grabbed me by the scruff of the neck and brought me back to life. He worked with me for a week 'in the field' as he liked to put it, often taking long drives into wilderness areas, visiting sites of potent geographical and historical significance, and even doing our work in a parking lot at Walgreens. His work was very unorthodox in the sense that all he was ever interested in was helping people reclaim their life force. If he had to throw you out of a plane with a parachute on your back for you to realise you were fully alive, that is what he would have done. He had this unorthodox way of working moment-to-moment with a person, in response to what they presented at the time. In this way, he gave me a blueprint for my work—which is, to have no blueprint at all.

For a number of years, I would fly to Montana and Ray and I would go into the wilderness and work together. Ray was a bit of a shaman, a sort of Carlos Castaneda character. He had that otherworldly quality, and yet at the same time if you passed him in the street, you might think he was a cowboy, just like any other from a ranch in Montana. I rarely speak of him, because it is hard to describe what he taught me without sounding somehow flaky or ridiculous or absurd, but the work I did with Ray was central to the strengthening of my core. This was what he felt to be the issue for me: I had a very fragile inner core that needed to be strengthened so I could go on and do what I wanted to do. Ray's credo was: loving, sharing, gifting. And that's how he believed that we should live our lives. To live life like this—loving, sharing, gifting—is radical. It indicates radical trust in the universe. When Ray was dying of cancer years later, the time came for the universe to give back to him. There was no holding back. People flew from all over the world to care for him. And when Ray died, it felt like every molecule in the universe was shimmering, and he was everywhere. The fact of his death somehow meant that his spirit of loving, sharing, gifting was everywhere. I felt closer to him, in some senses, after he died, but I miss him and I feel immensely grateful to him. Working with Ray helped galvanise my drive to continue the search and create a space for my own way of teaching.

## THE BREATH, THE FLOW OF LIFE

In the beginning, the kind of yoga I was doing was considered unorthodox, and possibly it still is. It was unorthodox in the sense that what I wanted to facilitate in my students was an understanding of life *moving through* the body, rather than the body being a little puppet that gets put into mechanical positions. I wanted my students to experience the organic life of the body ough the practice of yoga.

Through my work, I ask people to look at the doors that they have shut in themselves, to look at what is behind those doors. It's usually whatever is behind those closed doors that is going to bring freedom. Whatever we are refusing in ourselves, we are basically refusing in and from life. The first place to start is the breath.

In teaching, the essential discovery for me was the role of the breath. Very early on, what kept coming up was the way people shut down first by holding their breath. If you are holding your breath, you can't feel. And if you're holding your breath, you're refusing an experience, just like the little child who says, 'I'm going to hold my breath till I get that cookie'. It's a refusal. I began to see that the breath was absolutely central to untying the knots within. If you want to untie these knots, you have to start right in the middle of the person, which is their breath—their life force. The breath is either moving through the body or not moving through.

In my work, I take people through an extravaganza where I break down barriers. I deconstruct the blocks that are holding people back from feeling *in* the body. The work I do is not coercive or deliberately cathartic—I don't want to give that impression. I've no interest in wrenching open a door or forcing an opening. The essence of what I do is create a situation in which people feel safe enough and accepted enough and alive enough to open those doors if they're ready. Amazingly, people do open doors.

When I had people focus on making breath the priority, impeccable inner alignment was the consequence. Can you breathe freely? Can you feel your breath moving in your back? Students would arrive naturally at this beautiful inner alignment, which of course is what all the masters practised. How did

Iyengar discover what alignment was? He discovered it through feeling this life force moving through him, feeling where it moved clearly and where it didn't move clearly.

I kept discovering over and over again how it didn't work to puppeteer people, detail by detail, in these movements, because one hundred per cent of the time it resulted in people holding their breath. If you ask someone to make full, free breathing the *primary imperative* in every movement, it will lead to impeccable alignment. After so many years of being the authority, of telling students exactly where to put their arms and exactly how to hold their backs, that simple realisation just blew me away!

They say that we teach what it is that we most have to learn. No doubt there are doors within me that I have shut. And there are probably doors in me I'm not even aware that I've shut. I want to be a free and light and liberated person in my own self. Through working with people, I see the places in myself that need development. I see the aspects of myself that perhaps I'm refusing. For instance, when I work with someone, I might notice that I dislike that person's expression—I refuse it, or I criticise it, or I internally judge it. Because I'm a teacher, I have to stay with that feeling *and* stay with the person, I can't just walk away. It's a learning process for me, more than students can imagine.

As a yoga teacher I feel more and more that it is my job— and it's a lovely job to have—to be a presence for seeing people just as they are. We're all just dying to have someone see us as we are. People spend their whole life wanting someone who will see them so that they can say, 'I am loved'. When we say we're loved, what we are saying is that we have *been seen*. What we want seen is the soul of ourselves, the essence of ourselves, the core. It has nothing to do with being physically attractive, being sexy, earning this much money or living in that house. What we want is someone to see us for who we are. To love us for what we are. That's the common expression: 'I want someone who'll love me just as I am'.

When I work with someone, I'm just looking at the person. I am not trying to make them fit into a box, or a system, or even a movement principle. I am looking at where they are in that moment, and it's exciting because we take it from there. When people feel *seen* that way, they don't feel judged, they feel safe and accepted, and from that context we can start the work. There is no qualification to this acceptance—it's not 'once you get all fifty-two points of *trikonasana* you will be a good little yogi and I will think you're a good student'. We *begin* with the acceptance rather than assume that acceptance is something that will happen somewhere in the distant future.

Mahatma Gandhi said, 'Be the change that you want to see in the world'. If everybody wants to be seen, wants to be loved— and we could pretty accurately say that everybody does—then if I, as a practitioner, begin to see and accept myself as I really am—good, bad, warts and all—then I am also creating a space for anyone who is working with me to do similarly. It is a principle called 'resonance'.

When a teacher has more systems operating than a student, even just in a physical sense, that sets up 'resonance' in the room. If my fluid systems are operating, if my organs are operating, if my glands are flowing, if I'm living in all dimensions of my body, then that's resonating for me and in the room. Sometimes when a student is really knocked out by a particular bodily expression, or *asana* [physical posture], I might get right up against them, very close to their field, and start moving.

I might even take their hand so they can feel the movement through my body, and get them to feel the resonance that's coming through. It's a bit like if you take someone's hand and you start to skip along loosely when they're stiff; eventually either you're going to have to stiffen up or they're going to have to loosen up. And because I'm the teacher, it's the student who generally has to loosen up the way they're skipping. It's like picking up a rhythm or a physical expression of energy that a person might not have allowed before.

Much of the *asana* [physical posture] practice is about building up strength within the nervous system to sustain charge, however you want to qualify 'charge'—as movement of *prana* [life-force, energy] through the body; as intense feeling; or as stress. If you imagine increasing the flow of an electrical current through the body, that is what the *asana* practice and the *pranayama* [breathing] practices are doing. They are about making the vehicle of the body capable of sustaining this high level of charge—this equals living life to the fullest. *Asana* and *paranyama* practices are about cultivating the ability to feel and experience life and the whole range of its possibilities, without exception.

*Asana* means, literally, 'comfortable seat'. Each *asana*, or pose, is an expression of life: a tree, a bird, an insect, a foetus, a mountain, a sage, a child. When one enters an *asana*, it is a means of becoming comfortable in that expression of life. If there is something within me that is blocking that expression, then I'll come up against it in the course of my *asana* practice. When people are practising, they'll come across poses they absolutely hate—these are always the most interesting ones. There is something about that pose, that life expression that doesn't sit well in that particular individual. If a person works skilfully, and is being facilitated by a good teacher, then they'll work through whatever is blocking their expression. They'll be able to be the warrior in their life when they need to be the warrior, to be childlike when they need to be childlike, or to be quiet and still when they need to be quiet and still.

If you're not able to sustain those experiences without some kind of internal collapse going on, if you have a very low threshold for charge of any kind, then the moment something happens to you—whether it's a painful feeling or a pleasurable feeling or a stress in your job—you're going to shatter physically, psychically, emotionally and mentally. You're going to fracture. Through the practise of *asana*, you are increasing your ability to sustain higher and higher levels of charge, and to live more and more fully. Life therefore tends to get more intense, but it also becomes more joyous. It becomes both more joyous and, by definition, more painful, because the moment you say 'joy', there's the polarity to that: there is sorrow.

Generally the students who come to me wishing to work like this are those who have done exactly what I did. They've taken their yoga practice to the end of the line. They've dotted their i's and crossed their t's. Everything is in position and yet they're asking, 'Is this all there is?' And, 'Why hasn't my life changed?' 'Why am I coming up against the same problems over and over again in my relationships with others and with myself?' 'Why am I not happy?'

## SEARCHING FOR MORE

Twenty years ago when people telephoned yoga studios they had a vaguely correct idea of what yoga was. Now the most frequently asked question at the reception desk in Los Angeles is, 'Will I get a good workout?' This is a sad indictment of how our priorities have changed. Public perception in the west is that *asana*, from Hatha yoga, equals Yoga with a capital Y. That is unfortunate because *asana* is only a very small sliver of the yoga tradition and is only one of the eight limbs of the traditional practice (as described by Patanjali, the Indian sage who codified yoga in the *Yoga Sutras* around 200 BC). The eight limbs of classical yoga that Patanjali describes are about reminding us of our true nature. By focusing on just one limb to the neglect of the other seven, it is difficult to reach an understanding of our true inner nature. It is misleading for students to think that by doing this pose or that pose they will achieve a state of Yoga.

The eight limbs are hardly ever mentioned in a yoga class today, and, to be honest, they do not have to be discussed explicitly but can be made present in the room by the attitude and behaviour of the teacher. The *yamas* and *niyamas*, the first two of the eight limbs [which deal with moral observance and self-restraints], are the underpinnings of the whole practice of Yoga. They encompass an ethical code for living, in which one's relationship to others is as important as one's relationship to one's self. This might sound straightforward, but relationships are where most of us trip up in our lives. It does not matter one iota if you can get your feet on the back of your head if your relationships in the world are not balanced, loving or ethical. Early on in the *Yoga Sutras*, Patanjali says that if your mind is unclear, the best way you can realise yoga is to first clean up your relationships.

Relationships to others and relationships to one's self are the testing ground for all the other yogic practices. You might think you have it together, sitting on your meditation cushion, but you might be like the dog who is loving as long as his fur is stroked the right way: the moment someone brushes his fur the other way, he turns into a vicious attack animal. The practice is this: do your practice on your own but then test yourself in your relationship to the world. Test the soundness of your practice. That's what the *yamas* and *niyamas* are about: testing the soundness of your understanding that we are from the same source: what gives life to me also gives life to you. As Ray said, 'There are no strangers in this world.'

Patanjali gives four suggestions on how to cultivate ethical relationships. First, learn how to be peaceful with people who are already peaceful towards you. (That's not too hard.) Second, be friendly towards those who are suffering. (You'd think that might be easy too until you try it.) The third suggestion: take delight in another's happiness. The human mind is an interesting thing. There's a bumper sticker in New Zealand that says, 'Please God, if you can't make me thin, make everybody else fat'. We don't always celebrate when something good happens to other people, we often see it as a competitive threat, and it's only when bad things happen to other people that we can feel good about ourselves. Lastly, Patanjali says, practise tolerance or neutrality towards those who have harmed us or those who we dislike.

I remember when I first heard a talk given by Richard Freeman (an American ashtanga teacher who has trained extensively in eastern philosophy) in which he said, 'When we throw someone out of our heart it creates a hole in us. And only in returning that person back into our hearts will the hole heal.' I sat there thinking, 'Oh, what a wonderful thought,' and then, almost instantaneously, my mind suspected there had to be a loophole. There had to be a footnote in fine print somewhere that said, 'that is, except for your mother or your father-in-law, except for this person who has hurt me horribly, except for that person who pushes my buttons.' But the *Yoga Sutras* say that there are no exceptions. If we refuse some part of life, accordingly and to the same degree, we create separation within our selves.

*Asana* can help us realise this, but *asana* alone does not equal *yoga*. Because the western mind understands form, it has made the assumption that *asana* equals yoga. Hence the intent and purpose of yoga has been bastardised in the west in order to make it more palatable to the western mind, which wants security and certainty, and is concerned with form. The western mind can *understand* an object, but it cannot necessarily receive or value that which is *giving life* to the object. As a result, the focus of many yoga classes in the west has become body-fixated: practise yoga so you won't age, so you can have a beautiful body, so you can build up your abdominal muscles—all of these aims are a bastardisation of the original intent of yoga.

There is a well-known Zen trick where a Zen master takes a sheet of blank paper and sketches upon it the image of a bird, wings spread in flight. He holds it up in front of his students and asks the class what they see when they look at this drawing. The students reply: 'An eagle!' 'A seagull!' 'A bird!' The master considers their replies and then shakes his head. 'No,' he responds, 'It is a sky with a bird in it. You are only seeing the bird.'

The nature of the mind is that its attention is drawn to what is most salient—anything that is moving or loud or fragrant or sensory. But there is also a place from which all of these experiences arise. And yoga will take you there. People call this place the centre, the essence, or consciousness. I like to call it 'the natural mind'. With training, one can start to register this place and become able to exist simultaneously in both the world of the senses and the world beneath those senses.

The body, this form that seems so concrete, is part of who we are, but it's not all of who we are. If you think that your body is all of who you are, which is largely the western perspective, you are going to suffer terribly. The conundrum is that a spirit needs a body in which to exist. You have to have a body to have life force moving through it. The body is the medium for that current. The yogis were more aware than anyone that we mistake the body as the source of life, believing only that we are born, that we live and that we die. That is the fundamental error.

Yoga, in a very basic sense, is a practice for reminding oneself of that which is *giving* life. What is enlivening you? What is it that makes you alive? What is it that allows you to move that finger? What is it that creates the light behind your eyes? It is not you. It's this mystical, mysterious life force. Yoga is a practice we use to remind us of who we really are.

For me, *asana* has become almost an excuse for realising these other things. I happen to be a physical person. I happen to enjoy the body. If I were someone with a different proclivity I might have chosen to practise Bhakti yoga or Karma yoga [less physical forms of yoga]. I probably do practise Karma yoga [selfless action] as a teacher. It doesn't really matter what form of yoga you practise, the *asana* practice is important only in the sense that you have a direct felt experience. The truth of who we are can only be found through direct experience— anything else is just an intellectual understanding. The only way to have a direct felt experience is to be *in* the body. And if you're not in your body, if you think your body is something that carries your head around during the day, if you're disassociated from your body—and most people are extremely disassociated from their bodies—then you're disassociated from the source of your aliveness.

East or west, north or south, coast to coast, it doesn't matter what country I am in, I see this disassociation from the body happening all over the world. The reason is that the body is where we feel pleasure, but it is also where we feel pain. You don't get to choose. If you are going to be fully open to experiencing your life in your body, then you're going to feel pleasure and you're going to feel pain. You will experience sorrow and you will experience joy. If you don't have a threshold for the intensity of those sensations, then you may shut down your body so you feel neither pleasure nor pain.

The problem for most human beings is that they want certainty and they want security and if you are going to be fully alive you don't get either of those. They just don't go with the territory. If your main objective is to make life as secure and as certain as you possibly can—which is the impossible objective most of us spend the better part of our lives trying to achieve—then you're going to disconnect from many, many experiences that fall outside of the parameters of safety and security.

*Asana* practice won't change who you are fundamentally, but what it does do is open up your range of choices. If you start off neurotic, you're still going to be a little neurotic after years of your yoga practice. If you start off as a fearful person, you're probably going to be a fearful person later on in life in spite of practising yoga—but perhaps you will be fearful to a lesser extent.

I recognise, for instance, that I tend to be a fearful person, which surprises a lot of people. I tend to be a fearful person, but that does not stop me from going bareback-riding on my horse. That did not stop me from getting on an aeroplane on September 12. It doesn't stop me from doing those things because, through my yoga practice, I recognise my tendency to be fearful and am able to go behind it and beneath it to the place from which it arose. Are you able to recognise the bird in the sky, as the Zen master asks, and not just focus on the bird? Can you reside in the natural mind?

When we're deeply in touch with that place beneath the surface, the place that is untouched, the sub-stratum of whoever we are, then we can be living there. This is a confusing concept if you think that yoga is a personal development program, something you just get better at all the time, becoming more whole and, eventually, complete. The truth is that we are whole and complete to begin with.

The sub-stratum that lies beneath the outward manifestation of the Self is always there, and is absolutely intrinsic to our being. Even if we have been doing yoga for twenty years, and no matter how enlightened or masterful a person we are, there will still be a surface manifestation of our being. Even Ramana Maharishi, who was one of the most extraordinary yogis of this century, said he still felt emotions like everyone else feels— it's just that those feelings did not particularly bother him anymore. In other words, he existed in the sub-stratum. When people say to me, 'Oh, you do yoga, so you no longer feel any pain', I say, 'I feel pain like anybody else.' But because I am attempting, through my practice, to live in the sub-stratum of who I am, the place before there was any 'me', there is no 'I' to feel pain anymore, because that place is a pain-free place.

I know that yoga works, because it has worked for me. I say to my students that if it can work for me, if I can be a happy person who is alive in each moment, then it can work for anyone. When I look back at that sixteen-year-old girl who was living in such turmoil when she signed up for her first yoga class, I feel very grateful. I don't know if I'd be alive if I hadn't received a clear message right at that moment that I belonged in the universe. The ironic thing about being thrust from America to New Zealand and into a culture where I didn't fit is that it forced me to find the larger sense of where I belong. And through yoga I have found that.

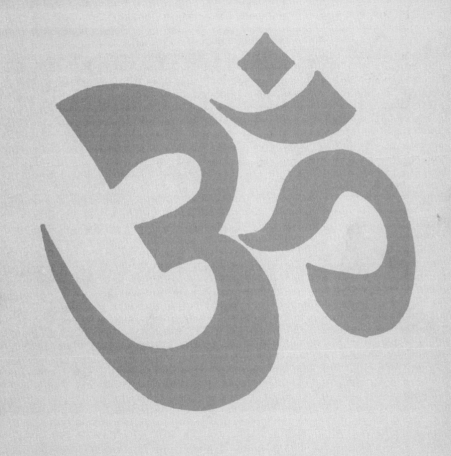

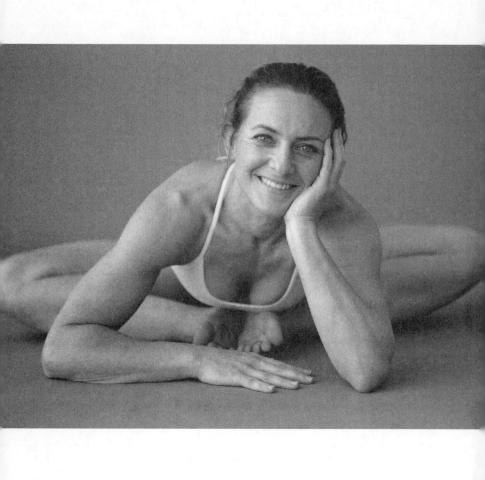

# 2

# EMBRACING LIFE

## *Eileen Hall*

*Practise, practise, all is coming.*

Sri K. Pattabhi Jois

*Running requires swiftness, speed, agility. Yoga: slowness, passivity, calm. At least that was the perception held by a young sprinter from Adelaide before she did her first yoga class. Now she is one of only a handful of ashtanga teachers in the world to be accredited to teach in the method of her guru, Sri K. Pattabhi Jois.*

*Eileen Hall was in her early twenties and a competitive track athlete when a friend handed her a newspaper advertisement for yoga at the local YMCA. She thought he must have been kidding. He wasn't and she went along. The appreciation and enjoyment she experienced was instant and set her on a new life path.*

*She began travelling regularly to India to study at the Ramamani Iyengar Memorial Yoga Institute, Pune, where she was accredited by B.K.S. Iyengar to teach Iyengar yoga. Then, on one trip, she made a second fateful decision. She dialled a telephone number scribbled onto a scrap of paper by another friend back home. The man who answered in Mysore, Sri K. Pattabhi Jois, became her teacher.*

*Jois was born on the full moon in July 1915. At the age of twelve he saw the great Hatha yogi, Professor T. Krishnamacharya (father of yoga author T.K.V. Desikachar and also teacher of B.K.S. Iyengar), give a demonstration and lecture, and approached him, requesting to become his student. He studied with Krishnamacharya for twenty-five years. He became a professor of Sanskrit and Advaita Vedanta at the Sanskrit College of Mysore. Today, Jois teaches ashtanga yoga with his grandson, Sharath Rangaswamy, at the Ashtanga Yoga Research Institute, Mysore. The ashtanga style of asana is taught in six set sequences and is so demanding that few proceed beyond the first. Upon his instruction, Eileen Hall opened her own studio, Ashtanga Yoga Moves, in Sydney in March 1996, where she continues the legacy and lineage of the ashtanga tradition.*

*Nearly fifteen years since their first meeting, Sri K. Pattabhi Jois is visiting Sydney on the final leg of his 2002 world tour. As a surprise*

*and a tribute to the man who she affectionately calls 'Guruji',
Eileen has transformed an art house cinema in East Sydney into
something of a shrine. Offerings of bright, luscious flowers drip
from the stage, plumes of heady fragrance rise from joss sticks to
purify the air, two swamis recite mantras and the squat elephant
god, Ganesha, keeps watch over the four hundred strong crowd.
The cinema screen flashes images of Jois's life: his eightieth birthday,
with his wife Amma, under a blessed shower of water; his first
trip to L.A., out of his dhoti and into trousers; teaching in Mysore
where he 'squashes' a student in a forward bend; as he is now,
the Brahmin thread draped around his chest, three white stripes
across his brow and his caramel-coloured skin touched lightly
by time.*

*Legs in lotus, ever-smiling, Eileen talks about how she found
her teacher, her faith in him, and what was required in order to
establish a spiritual school in a material world.*

## RUNNING TO STAND STILL

Several years ago, in India, I went to see a Vedic astrologer
named Shankara, who practises *Jyotisha* [Vedic astrology].
He looked at my chart and I asked him, 'Shankara, what
do you see in my chart? Will I be a yoga teacher?' He
answered immediately, 'Yes, this is your destiny. It is your
higher purpose in this life!'

Since I was eight years old, I had been a competitive
athlete. When I turned twenty, I moved from Adelaide to
Sydney, where I met a friend who asked me if I had tried
yoga. I looked at him askance. 'I don't do yoga, I am a
sprinter!'

Like most people, I held a misinformed notion from pictures I had seen in books that yoga was about sitting still for long periods of time, and I knew that was not for me. I needed to move, to be active. This friend of mine, however, wasn't deterred. Persisting, he handed me a small advertisement for a six-week yoga course at the YMCA that he had cut out of the local newspaper. I relented and signed up.

The teacher was Ursula Trumpold, an Iyengar instructor. I remember there were about ten other women in the class, all of whom wore black leotards and were well over forty-five. In these humble surroundings, I fell in love with yoga. I finished one course and signed up for the next. During my fourth course, Ursula approached me and said, 'I want you to take over the class. I am going to India.'

I didn't refuse, but was somewhat overawed about teaching something I had only just been introduced to myself. I prepared by reading some yoga books and purchasing the necessary equipment: belts, straps and bolsters. The first class came along and, although nervous, I applied myself to teaching, engaged with the students, and found I loved it. About a month later, Ursula returned and simply said, 'Now I will take you to my teacher.'

She took me to Robert Lucas, who was one of the first *ashtanga* yoga teachers in Australia. Robert was a surfie, with sun-bleached hair, a long blond beard and a resemblance to Jesus. Tall and lean, he hardly spoke a word. There were just three of us in the room and he guided us through our practice, flowing through the poses, one into the next. I felt an immediate and heartfelt connection with this style of yoga. I went along the next Saturday, and the next—I never missed one—and then on the fourth Saturday, Lucas was gone. He had disappeared, left without notice, gone walkabout, as yogis do. But at our third session, he had told me a little bit about his teacher, an Indian man called Pattabhi Jois, and had given me his phone number in Mysore.

Over the next two years I continued practising and teaching yoga, travelling to Pune, where I was certified to teach by B.K.S. Iyengar. Studying with Iyengar was remarkable. He is an incredibly passionate, committed and dedicated person: a true genius. But after a while I felt something was missing in my practice in the Iyengar style. I felt like I was taking out an instrument and tuning it—bing, bing, bing—but never really getting to strum the chords. I became disillusioned with Iyengar yoga's rigid form, so on one of my trips to Pune, I called up Pattabhi Jois and asked him if I could come to Mysore and study with him.

On our first meeting, we bonded instantly. It felt as though I had stepped into my destiny. Walking into the room, seeing Pattabhi Jois, I had a strong feeling that this was all meant to be. I was coming home. I knew I had found my teacher.

Pattabhi Jois's own teacher, Professor T. Krishnamacharya, was also B.K.S. Iyengar's teacher and one of the first Indian gurus to agree to teach westerners, particularly women. I knew this, and so when I first visited Pattabhi Jois I came with an appreciation of this history. Krishnamacharya broke tradition and was frowned upon for doing so, but it's a blessing that he did. Had he conformed to tradition, yoga wouldn't be where it is now in the west. As yoga's popularity grows, it's important to acknowledge its integrity but to let the tradition be flexible and open.

In the early eighties only a handful of people went to India, and they were largely considered crazy for going all the way to a small village in the middle of nowhere to study with a teacher who back then was little known. There wasn't a website, or a map, and there wasn't a *Yoga Journal* directory. You had to ask people, 'Where is he?' Someone would say, 'I have heard he is in Mysore somewhere.' But it was in making this journey that something invaluable occurred. It gave me an opportunity to face my fears and answer my own doubts about what I was doing, why I was going there. By the time I arrived I was ready to embrace the unknown and commit to my practice.

In those days, there were no casual classes—you had to study for a minimum of three months. Nor was there email to stay in touch with family and friends back home, you had to put your career on hold or abandon it altogether. There was a sense of isolation from the outside world and its values—this created an intensity that was ultimately empowering.

It has now become universally accessible to study yoga with a guru in India. You can search for Pattahbi Jois's address on the website, download it, print it out, complete with bus routes and instructions on where to stay and how to find breakfast after morning practice, down the laneway, at Nagaratna's kitchen. It is easy now and because of that, the intensity has eased and less commitment is required. Some students go because they are curious, some are shopping around, and others go because it is considered fashionable to practise yoga with an Indian guru.

In the early days, though, students surrendered themselves totally to the guru. It went unquestioned. Now students ask questions: why does he charge so much money? why does he do what he does? When you go to study yoga there with an attitude that the guru needs to prove himself, then you are blocking yourself with your own preconceived ideas. When you are in the presence of someone who can teach you something about yourself, open yourself up and let go of expectations and preconceptions. Like an empty cup, you let the guru fill you up. If you go in there already half full, he has to tip out the contents first. Some people don't like doing that, because what the guru is challenging is their self-identity.

## OPENING THE HEART

On my first day of yoga practice with Pattabhi Jois, he sat with me and chuckled. 'You step! You step!' he kept repeating. I would reply, 'With which leg?' And he would laugh. After fifteen minutes, he stopped me, sat with me, and took me through some breathing exercises, which is a very important aspect of *ashtanga* yoga. We did that for three weeks.

One afternoon, on the second week of my stay, I felt an incredible fever wash over me. I went to bed and wound a wet scarf around my head to relieve the throbbing pressure behind my eyes. My body fluctuated between being blistering hot and freezing cold. I lost all sense of time and space and stayed in this state for two days, before a friend, thinking I had contracted malaria or typhoid, took me to see a doctor. The doctor was nonplussed. Growing more anxious about my condition, my friend sought Pattabhi Jois's help. Guruji's response was: 'In three days, all right.'

Sure enough, after three days I woke up as if nothing had happened. I went to class the next day and Guruji was smiling. 'Okay now?' he asked me. I began to tell him just how sick I had been, half expecting sympathy, but what he said instead touched me more deeply. 'Ahhh,' he said, with understanding in his voice, 'heart is opening.'

In that moment my appreciation of the practice transformed. I understood that there are many subtle levels and layers that yoga can affect. I learnt a big truth that day and was able to surrender to the depths of yoga.

The last trip to India was my twenty-third. I went to Pune perhaps five or six times initially to study with the Iyengar family, and ever since I have been going to Mysore to study with Pattabhi Jois. It was perhaps at the end of my fourth trip to Guruji, when I stayed for six months, that he asked me, 'Where you going?' I said, 'I am going back to Sydney.' He said, 'Go to Sydney and set up one school and you teach.'

There are only a handful of teachers in the world to whom Guruji has given his blessings to teach. I didn't go to Mysore with that intent; I went there to understand more about myself. Now I was to become a teacher.

## YOGA IN ANOTHER FORM

I didn't have any experience in business and this was a huge burden for me when I started the school. When most people were getting ahead in their jobs, I was travelling back and forth to India. What I learnt about running the business side of the school is that business is yoga in another form. It is about patience, it is about peeling away the layers, and it is about learning to communicate with staff in a yogic way. When I write a cheque, do I write it with the same integrity that I use in adjusting someone's pose? Is there a difference? There is yoga in everything we do; it is about acting with mindfulness and in a heart-felt way. Every student is unique, whether advanced or beginner. They are all on a journey, and for part of it, I am their guide.

Combining the traditional practice with the business side of running a yoga school remains a constant challenge. At times I don't know whether to open the *Bhagavad Gita* or my cheque-book, and it's then I ask the guru for help. If I am ever in doubt, I always ask him. And his answers are always very simple. Usually, 'Only God knows.' By this he means, literally, only God knows our destiny and it will unfold accordingly.

Whenever I visit Mysore, I still get an urge to stay. Part of me feels more at home in India with Guruji. As soon as I get there, a big sigh leaves my body. I feel the comfort of the temperature, the warmth of the people who love the practice I love. Some days, particularly when they're rough, I ask myself, 'Why are you living in Sydney when you could be in India?' But my guru has told me that I am a westerner and India is not my home; my home is back in the west and that's where I should be teaching.

To go to India to live would be comfortable, but when you are comfortable you can get very *tamasic*, very dreary and stale in your body and spirit. Wherever I am, I know that I'm never far from the spirit of yoga, from my guru, or from India. I can embrace all of that in simple ways like lighting a candle or a stick of incense. The challenges of bringing yoga to the west are always enriching—they stoke the inner fire and ignite the spirit. For me these things are found here now, in Sydney, teaching at my school.

Unfortunately, the more people yoga reaches, the more people view it solely on the physical level without understanding the depths of the practice. The physical practice *does* give stress relief, it *does* help an aching back, it *will* quieten the mind and free the breath, and all these physical benefits serve us immensely and instantly—you can feel it from the very first class you do. But if you really want to penetrate to the heart of the practice, you will need to touch on that which Patanjali describes in the *Yoga Sutras*: yoga is all about the mind.

There is little in the *Yoga Sutras* that tells us about *asana*; instead the *Yoga Sutras* is focused on the breath and the mind. A lot of people don't want to engage with this deeper aspect of yoga, because it can be very confronting. They are happy to stay on the surface and to work with the form that we see when we hold up a mirror. But it is the form you don't see reflected in the mirror that comes to the surface when you are working closely with a teacher. You begin to work much deeper than just physically, and the teacher is able to see where your strengths lie and where your weaknesses hide, and can work with those distinctions. When I build up a relationship with a student, some days they can look like a Dalmatian. I can see spots over their body where they are holding on, where they are not letting go, where the breath is not flowing. You wonder to yourself, why is that happening? What are they holding onto and why are they not letting the *prana*, the life force, flow?

Surrendering and opening up on deeper levels comes with time. It comes with breathing and with letting the heart open. There are so many things that we push away from our heart, and that inner resistance creates our anger, our fears and our discomfort. To be whole and happy we need to bring those things back into our heart. The heart is the place of no conditions, no expectations, unconditional love and total acceptance, but it is really hard for human beings to safeguard this space as sacred. Most of us hold onto expectations and conditions, especially when it comes to our relationships with others and with ourselves, and when these expectations or conditions get broken we discover where our illusions lie.

The first time I went to Mysore there were just three of us in the *shala*. When Guruji had only a handful of students, he could bond with each of us—now he has hundreds, and he might see students for four weeks and then never see them again. You can teach someone the *asana*, but to really understand their shadows, you need to know more about them and that doesn't come just by going to someone once a week for six weeks—that comes with time. The word *guru* means someone who takes you from darkness to light, from your shadows to your inspiration.

It is my belief that what is happening on the physical plane is a reflection of what is happening on an emotional and psychological plane. From day to day, I see in my students a totally different body. How can the body be so different from one day to the next? It is our thoughts that create that difference. Therefore, thoughts have to change, otherwise the body won't shift. If your thinking doesn't change, then you just keep repeating old patterns. That is another reason why working with a teacher is necessary: it prevents us from creating an illusion of who we think we are. The teacher will take you from darkness to light and help you see where you are hiding in the shadows. No matter how much you twist, sweat and grunt, and turn yourself inside out, if your heart is not in the practice, if your spirit is not there, then changing your body won't make any difference to your psyche. For real change to take place, the heart must be willing.

Cultivating mindfulness and integrity in your practice—and then learning to apply those same qualities to life—is the art of yoga. When you approach your practice, surrender into it and have no expectation of the outcome. Then you can roll up your mat, walk out of the yoga room, and continue to be present and openhearted and without expectation with your lover and with your family, with your colleagues, and with your environment. That is how yoga can transform the whole of your life, not only your body.

## ALL PATHS LEAD HOME

A lot of people question what style of yoga is best. The different styles of yoga simply cater to different personalities. When you start to understand that, you realise that yoga is universal; it is a practice for everyone. All forms of yoga share a collective belief and are based on a universal concept of union, which manifests in a deep, heart-felt experience of being alive. As Deepak Chopra explains, human souls have incredible potential and yoga is one tool to release that potential, to let go of what scares us, to surrender and to be inspired.

People think yoga is *trikonasana* [triangle pose] and backbending, but really the poses are about bringing our body and our mind back into a state of balance. Hatha yoga, to use the umbrella term for styles of yoga that emphasise the practice of *asana* (including *ashtanga*), is about bringing the energies of the sun and the moon back into balance in order to steady the mind. The various postures act to heat or to cool the body until you become just the breath. When you align the opposing heating and cooling energies of the sun and the moon, when you steady the breath, then you can begin to work with the practice of meditation. The quality of your breath is an indication of the state of your mind: if the breath is fluctuating, then you can guarantee that the mind is unsteady as well. The *asanas* are therefore a tool to ultimately steady the mind. This is the great gift of yoga to the west and a reason for its popularity.

B.K.S. Iyengar once said to me: 'One student coming, I am thanking God. No student coming, I am thanking God.' By this, he meant that he either had an opportunity to share the yoga with others, or he had time to practise himself. For me, that's what it comes down to. Gratitude. If one person turns up to your class, be grateful. And for westerners, you don't just turn up to a class, you have to think about it the night before. People have to pack their bag and get organised beforehand— in this way, their thought of coming to your class has actually started twelve hours earlier.

I see everyone who comes into the yoga studio as trying to become a better person—that's why he or she comes to class. If you have that very simple attitude as a teacher, then the teaching comes easily. And the teacher doesn't only teach something to the student; there is an interrelationship between the two. If you have difficulty relating to a student, you will find that it is an indication of something in yourself that you are not embracing or not seeing. To be totally accepting of all people means that you are totally accepting of everything within yourself.

Guruji embodies this spirit of acceptance. He will teach the practice to anyone who walks in his door. He places no judgement on anyone. Everyone he encounters is a pure being, a pure light. There is a concept of destiny and purpose in his teaching that goes beyond the physical world. He embodies a spiritual vision of spreading the understanding of yoga. It is his duty to teach. That's what he believes. And I think that, beyond duty, he teaches because it is a love—a love of God and a love of all existence, all sentient beings.

Pattabhi Jois is nearly ninety and he doesn't tire. He teaches every day, starting before dawn and finishing by lunchtime. He performs his duties with a profound understanding of the universal purpose of his being and his responsibility to humankind in passing on wisdom.

I spoke to Guruji just the other day because it was *Guru Poornima*, the festival to celebrate and honour your guru. I rang him up in Mysore and he said to me, 'Why you not here?' I replied, 'Guruji! I was only just there!' I had visited Mysore several weeks earlier. The *ashtanga* community is like a family, which Pattabhi Jois nurtures—he is the strength and the core of it, and the loving sense of family radiates from him. You can go anywhere in the world, from Paris to New York, and if you practise at the *ashtanga* school, someone will always ask you to say 'hi' to their friend who you may know. It's a network that has developed, like a fine web connecting us all over the world. In the same way that Guruji has created a sense of the *ashtanga* community-as-family, his own family is very important to him. When he travels to teach, his immediate family travel with him.

He made his fourth trip to Australia recently. The first time he visited I was nervous—what do you do with an Indian Brahmin? How do you entertain him? Do you take him to the movies? What does he eat? Where does he stay? I learnt that you just relax. And if you don't know, you ask. Guruji stays in a hotel with his family because his daughter Saraswati does the cooking. He is a Brahmin and the custom is that a Brahmin will only eat food from a banana leaf prepared for him by another Brahmin.

On his first trip, after picking Guruji up from the airport, we took him to see the school, Yoga Moves, which he had never seen before. At the top of the steps we had a statue of Ganesha [the Elephant God who removes obstacles]—unbeknown to us, its position in the room was totally unacceptable because it was right next to where you remove your shoes. In India, you don't walk in front of a deity with your shoes on, let alone remove them and leave them lingering in front of a sacred being. Guruji looked around the space, 'Move him there!' So we moved him to where we were instructed, beneath the eastern windows where the light floods in. Months later several students who practise the Chinese art of *feng shui* confirmed that Ganesha was now in the most auspicious space in the room.

Guruji first travelled to the west in 1974 in order to understand better how westerners live and think—which is very different to how an Indian perceives life. This has enabled him to understand why we manage relationships the way we do—he couldn't understand that before. He would say, 'Last year you come with this man. Now you come with that man. What happened?'

Indian tradition usually demands that you are married for life, and Guruji had a very loving relationship with his wife, Amma, who is no longer alive. As he has opened up to the west and seen first-hand how we live and think, the yoga practice he teaches has changed a lot. Students who went to him twenty years ago will tell you that the practice was totally different back then—over time, his teaching has evolved into a more accessible form.

Things have also changed in Mysore. Guruji has moved on from the old *shala* [yoga studio], which was originally his family home too. The old *shala* was sold to the bank! I thought that was a shame because there was a lot of history in that room. The new *shala* opened in 2002. The opening ceremony was a fantastic celebration. A lot of Guruji's older students were there, including Eddie Stern, a long-time American student and teacher, who produced a booklet with the actress and *ashtanga* practitioner Gwyneth Paltrow that documents Guruji's life in pictures and words. Eddie has been a musician in New York for years and he arranged for a famous Indian musician, Anup Jalota, to sing *bhajans* at the opening ceremony. It was like having George Harrison in your living room. When Eddie told Guruji that this musician was flying in from Bombay, Guruji was thrilled—and his grandson, Sharath, couldn't speak for excitement. All the residents of the neighbourhood poured onto the street, trying to rubberneck and see Anup Jalota, but the *shala* was only open for the students to preview.

The official opening was held the next day with the traditional *homas*, the fire ceremonies that clear the spirits and create the energies of the school. A procession of Brahmin priests started at the top of the *shala* and proceeded through each room, so that by the time they got to the bottom floor the place was one hazy smoke zone. The only people left indoors were the priests and Guruji. Everyone else was smoked-out, tears streaming and coughing. Guruji was running after us, unperturbed, saying, 'Come! You come!'

Later that night Guruji said to me, 'Eileen, what think you?'

I thought. 'Your vision was to create a big, beautiful centre where students could come,' I said. 'Now you are eighty-eight and you have done it. You have followed your dream. This is an inspiration for us all.'

He replied, 'Not my school, Sharath's school.'

'It is your school too,' I said. 'You built this.'

'No. I am old man. Sharath's castle now.'

'You are not old, Guruji! Teaching all the students keeps you young.'

'Correct!' he beamed. 'Eighty-eight years old now. Upon completing class, feeling sixty-eight!'

Guruji's love for what he does and his sense of purpose towards mankind keeps him young. I have deep gratitude that such a man is my teacher. It is said that when the student is ready the teacher will appear. Without knowing it, I must have been ready thirteen years ago when I picked up the phone and asked to study with him. I knew that this was a great man who could teach me a lot about yoga, but I didn't anticipate that he would also teach me so much about love.

On Guruji's last visit to Sydney, we surprised him with a tribute night in his honour. All his students came, new and old. It was an incredible party and it gave me the chance to show my gratitude. In front of everyone present that night I said: 'Thank you, Guruji, for allowing me to be your student. Thank you, Guruji, for sharing your life and the spirit of yoga with the humility that only a great guru can. You opened my eyes to realise the depth and mystery of yoga, and to appreciate the power of this practice to open the hearts of human existence. I thank you and I bow before you.'

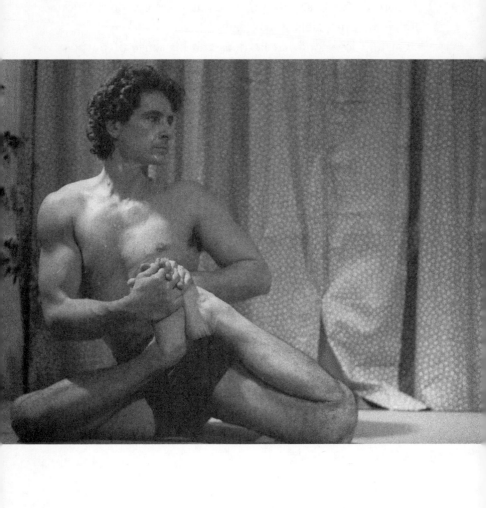

# 3

# LIVING FROM THE HEART

## *Glenn Ceresoli*

*Whatever I am offered in devotion with a pure heart — a leaf, a flower, fruit, or water — I accept with joy.*

Bhagavad Gita

When Glenn Ceresoli's girlfriend asked him to sign up for a yoga class in 1979, he dismissed the idea of yoga as something better suited to out-of-shape housewives. The then nineteen-year-old was more interested in pumping weights, playing rock guitar and racing his motorcycle around the streets of Melbourne. But his girlfriend was keen that they do something together as a couple, and reluctantly he agreed.

From a young age Glenn excelled at whatever activity he attempted, be it bodybuilding, martial arts, running, cycling or soccer. His physical prowess was obvious. But when Glenn was ten years old, his father died, prompting an inner questioning that no physical activity could provide the answers for. He applied himself to every new challenge with a relentless vigour that he hoped would take him beyond his boundaries and open up new understandings. Nothing did.

In that initial yoga class, the one he begrudgingly attended, the answers began to come. Something shifted. Yoga challenged him physically and satisfied him inwardly, and it became his obsession. In 1983, he met Shandor Remete, who taught him Iyengar yoga. By 1986, Glenn was given the responsibility of running The Action School of Yoga in Melbourne.

But yoga proved to be both his salvation and his downfall. There were potholes on the road ahead and he fell into them. Success was one; obsessiveness was another. He was too busy nurturing the school to nurture his family; his marriage suffered. Despite being a master on the mat, his priorities off it were confused.

For all the external efforts Glenn made in yoga, he realised that what needed to change was within him. He left his successful school, packed up and moved away from the city. He peeled back the layers of ego, ambition and obsession, dismantled the scaffolding that upheld his idea of himself, and began to search for the core of who he truly was. What he learnt was that composure on the mat cultivated composure in life, right intention brought about right action. For true happiness you must find the heart, which is the centre of who you are.

Glenn has a thick mop of dark curls that are faintly dusted grey— a telltale sign of his pitta [fiery] nature. His eyes shine like black polished stone and his trademark t-bar goatee underlines an often wry smile. His body testifies to its rigorous Iyengar training: symmetrically proportioned, graceful and strong. Twenty-odd years of asana have erased all trace of his bulky body builder past. Glenn's right hand fingernails are long and coated with acrylic, hardened enough in order to pluck the strings of his beloved acoustic guitar. On the middle finger of his right hand sits a knuckle-duster of a gold ring, set with a rectangle of black onyx and bordered by glinting diamonds, a gift for Glenn from Satya Sai Baba, the well-known Indian guru who is said to be a divine incarnation and who possesses the supernatural ability to make objects manifest. To look at Glenn now there is no sign of the anger, no sense of the ill ease that once dogged him and forced a radical life change.

He lives now with his wife Margaret and their two young sons, Jai and Jordan, at the foot of Mount Warning, an extinct volcano on the eastern seaboard of Australia. When he is not touring the world giving demonstrations, workshops and intensives, or assessing teachers for the B.K.S. Iyengar Yoga Association of Australia, he is planting trees on the property, collecting his sons from the bus stop after school and rekindling his love for the guitar. It is a world far removed from the one he left behind. Here Glenn talks about why he needed to leave the life he was living in order to reconnect with his centre.

## PUSHING THE LIMITS

At eighteen, I started running around Melbourne's Princess Park to get my fitness up. The first time I ran halfway around, stopped and drove home. As I was driving I asked myself, 'Why did I stop?' I didn't know. So when I returned the next day I decided to run all the way around. I didn't die. It was easy enough. I felt a bit sore but not enough to stop. I was still stuck on the question though: What makes me stop?

The following day I decided to keep running until I knew what caused me to stop. After a few laps I was feeling tired but I knew that I could go further so I sprinted. I kept running around and around until I eventually eased myself to a jog— otherwise I could have kept going. I realised that the desire to stop was not coming from my body, but from my mind.

This taught me an important lesson: there are no limits. We might think we have to 'Stop!', but there is always more capacity, energy and potential than what we limit ourselves to. We limit ourselves because of preconceived ideas, convenience or comfort. We consider an action to require too much effort and don't bother. The ability to *do*, and the potential within us, is always greater than we think. Running taught me this and it then became an underlying theme in my life. When I started yoga I always thought, 'Why stop now? There must be more there.' Constantly pushing my limits allowed me to discover deeper aspects of myself, and this opened up a new world of possibilities.

From my early teens I took part in all sports and usually excelled, but the idea of being the best wasn't enough. I felt an inner urge for 'more' but I was too young to understand what this was. I tried other forms of sport that also demanded mental concentration, like martial arts, but I never found the right teacher. In hindsight, I know that what I was looking for was a teacher who was not motivated by ego or monetary gain but by a sincere intention to teach the traditional values which embody the spirituality of martial arts.

At nineteen years old I was pushing weights, and the full bodybuilding mentality had kicked in. Previously I had been a junk food king. I used to eat anything and everything and five times more than I needed. When I got serious about bodybuilding I started to watch my diet, reading nutrition books, measuring calories, vitamins and minerals. This made me aware of a new aspect of performance—which gave me an edge.

In my pursuit of 'the edge', I got quite fanatical about what I consumed. I documented everything I put into my mouth and analysed it each night. I completely removed the sensual pleasure of food and took in only what was essential. I reached a physical high where I would go to bed at night and not be able to sleep because my body was vibrating. I was running on nervous energy and could only sleep for four to five hours, but I felt fantastic. Again I thought, 'Why stop? Why go back to eight hours sleep if I feel fantastic on four?' Soon I was losing too much weight, I was feeling too 'light' and I realised my behaviour was perhaps bordering on the extreme.

At this stage in my life, working out at the gym and playing rock music were my passions. My dream was to become a rock guitarist. My father had been a part-time musician and had named me after the Big Band leader, Glenn Miller. My girlfriend at the time was looking for something for us to do together. She suggested we do an eight-week yoga course. It was like offering tofu to a meat-eater. I told her, 'Yoga is not for me! I need something with grunt.'

My initial resistance was due to ignorance and a strong male ego that rejected anything 'wimpy'. I had always been ambitious in whatever activities I undertook, be it raging on the weekend or running around an oval. The desire to move beyond my limits was always there, and I needed it in order to feel a deeper sense of who I was. I did not think yoga could offer me that. I also had an inbuilt anti-religious attitude due to childhood experiences.

When I was eight years old my family moved to Italy. Six months later my mother returned to Australia for work. My father was too ill to look after me so I was sent to Catholic boarding school. The hypocrisy I saw in the caretaker's and priest's behaviour—preaching one thing and behaving differently—made me wary of anything with a religious tag, which in my mind included yoga.

My girlfriend persisted and I gave in. I justified my change of mind by reasoning that yoga was just a set of harmless stretches. I also remembered what I had learnt from running: there was greater potential beyond what I knew. I should at least open my mind to that possibility.

On the first night of the course at the Integral School of Yoga in Melbourne, I noticed a strange smell when we opened the door. It was incense. I looked around and I could see framed images of a swami! We went into the room and there was an altar! Alarm bells went off. I was searching for the exit. I kept reminding myself to keep an open mind. If I didn't like it, I didn't have to come back.

The stretching and poses relieved some of my muscular tightness from weightlifting, then to finish we did *savasana* [corpse pose—complete bodily relaxation] and then something happened. The yoga must have opened up or activated some energy centres within me because when I lay down I experienced something I had never felt before. What I know now is that I went into an expanded state of consciousness. I wanted to explore this further and eagerly went back the next week. The short story is that my girlfriend stopped, and I kept going. I felt that my thirst for an 'unknown something' that had eluded me since my early teens was finally being quenched.

This was it! This was what I had been looking for. I started buying books about the philosophy of yoga and practising the poses at home. The more I read and practised, the more yoga provided a philosophical outlook that opened up my mind beyond the boundaries that had confined me. The teachings of Swami Satchidinanda, who was the esteemed head of the Integral School of Yoga, were very pragmatic. He had the ability to bring abstract philosophy into the practical reality of how you lived your everyday life. This was very important to me.

What attracted me to *asana* practice [the practice of physical postures] was that it allowed me to measure where I was at and how real my experience was. The experience was not only in my head but became a *part* of me. Due to its inner process, *asana* allows for greater reflection and demands that you are present in the moment. In our age of sensual gratification and physical prowess, there is always a risk that you will end up further lost in *maya*, the illusory world of who you *think* you are. Without the necessary inner enquiry, *asana* degenerates to an exercise or stretching program.

I started to get up at five in the morning, shower, go through the *mantras* and *slokas* [Sanskrit verses from a prayer or hymn] and meditate. I would then do the sequence of *asanas* I learnt at Integral Yoga. That was the start of my day, every day. Afterwards I'd go to work at the gym, which I managed and where I would do my weights workout. At night, I would do my *asana* practice and a short meditation before going to bed.

My mum would come home to find me on the floor in all sorts of positions with incense wafting through the house.

'What the hell are you doing?' she'd ask.

'It's yoga, Mum,' I'd reply.

One day she came home and said, 'I don't understand what it is you do with this yoga, but whatever it is I like it and I approve. I have seen a positive difference in you over the last six months. You've made big changes to your attitude and the way you behave and this tells me that whatever you're doing is good.' That was a big confirmation for me.

Within one year, the Integral Yoga sequence was no longer challenging me. My enthusiasm for the *asana* practice was waning. Just as I was questioning my interest, I received this affirmation. One day I was driving to the beach with a friend and we were talking about different philosophical approaches to life. He started talking about something I was aware of but hadn't considered in depth: reincarnation. Tears started to well up in my eyes. They weren't due to sadness but to a recollection of an absolute truth about the transient nature of existence that I had long forgotten. I understood then that where I was and who I was was a culmination of all that I had done in the past. I understood that I needed to learn certain lessons. At that moment I felt compelled to continue with what I had been doing. I knew I was on the right track.

A short time later I met with a severe motorbike accident. My knee was badly injured and the doctors told me I would need a knee reconstruction, but my friend suggested I go to see his teacher, Shandor Remete, for yoga therapy. I went along before class to talk to him about my knee and he said something like, 'Take your shirt off and do the class.' I did the class, which was more intense than what I had done before, and immediately knew this was the yoga I was looking for. *Asana* became my priority. I didn't want anything to hinder my progress, so in time I stopped working out in the gym.

One evening I was leaving class when Shandor said to me, 'Have you ever considered dedicating your life to this, I think you would be good at it.' I dismissed the idea at the time. A month or so later I asked Shandor what would be required of me to start teaching. I began practising with him in the mornings and assisting in the evenings, and not long after that he gave me a 10 a.m. class to teach. I jumped in the deep end and swam. Though uncertain and nervous about what I was doing, I wasn't deterred. Often only one or three people turned up to my class, never more than four. Shandor would be at the back of the room doing his practice, which sometimes distracted the students, and I would have to draw their attention back to what I was instructing them to do.

Shandor never really had a lot to say to me. He never needed to. I was already trying as hard as I could. He saw that there were certain qualities in me and he allowed them to flourish. I never succeeded in finding a music teacher or a martial arts instructor who I clicked with, but Shandor's passion for what he did and his sense of commitment and conviction towards yoga was obvious. We got on very well.

We practised together in the mornings, and at one stage we were doing a lot of backbends, which were exciting. I disliked forward bends, because I found them too passive. It took me three years to do a decent forward bend, because I was reluctant to challenge those areas that were less pleasing to me. We started doing backflips (*viparita chakrasana*), where you inhale, exhale, drop back into a backbend, flip your legs over and land on your feet, inhale, take two steps forward, exhale and drop back again. We did one hundred and eight in twenty-two minutes, then something happened to my back. I was on my way to teach a class and I collapsed in the back laneway. I dragged myself up the stairwell and by the time I reached the class I had found the inner resolve to stand up and teach as if nothing had happened. To me, any pain was a sign that I was breaking through a limitation. I didn't have enough experience to know the difference between a damaging pain and a constructive pain. As I would soon discover, this was a damaging pain.

As a result of my motorcycle accident one knee was very different from the other, which was causing irregularity in my pelvis and therefore my spine. After months of doing these backflips and other advanced backbends, I had to curl my knees up to my chest to roll out of bed, and then crawl on my hands and knees to the door handle so I could stand up. Then I would get on my mat and start to undo the damage. The damage was caused by a combination of things: my refusal to do forward bends, the imbalance created from my knee and being excessive with my yoga practice. This marked the start of a two-year rehabilitation period that taught me what is a fundamental principle of yoga. It taught me not to just go with my favoured poses but to move beyond the likes and dislikes of the mind in order to attain balance in the body and mind.

In 1986, Shandor left Melbourne and offered me the school, which I relocated to Fitzroy as the Action School of Yoga. Not only was I unknown as a teacher, but yoga, back then, was also unknown. Nobody understood how it could help. A motto I came up with and still use today is: 'Whatever you do, yoga can help you to do it better.' The postures give you a fitter vehicle by affecting the muscles, joints, glands and the nervous system. Yoga teaches you to keep your calm. It gives you confidence and strength in the face of extreme situations. It requires you to hone your ability to focus and to develop the capacity to enquire and internally assess yourself and your circumstances clearly. Any endeavour you aspire to do well requires the same skills that are cultivated through yoga.

The mission for the Action School of Yoga was to establish credibility for yoga in the mainstream. To achieve this objective, I spread myself widely. I took classes at educational institutions, dance studios, martial arts schools. I would take lunchtime and private classes, even teaching at a fancy hairdressing salon. Once I took a workshop at a residential martial arts school. It was held in a basketball court and I was surrounded by a sea of two hundred and fifty heads, more students than I'd ever seen before. They weren't the slightest bit interested in yoga. I got an idea and said, 'Listen, you guys like doing high kicks. Then you want to be able to do this.' I spontaneously dropped to the floor into the side splits (*samakonasana*). 'Or this.' Front splits (*hanumanasana*). Their jaws hit the floor. All of a sudden they were into it, and anytime I'd fire off an instruction they would respond in a guttural '*Hai!*'.

That same year my relationship with Margaret, who is now my wife, started to develop. Two years later came the birth of our first child, Jai. I was still focused on getting the school off the ground and had many conflicting responsibilities and ambitions: a fledgling business needs nurturing, as does a young family. Then we had our second son, Jordan. All of these demands were difficult to blend together. On top of everything else, music re-entered my life. Although it had always been my dream, I had left music behind when yoga swept me off my feet.

I was trying to be a husband, and a father to two small boys, attempting to establish a credible school, teaching from six in the morning and rehearsing with my band until 1 a.m. most nights. When the band started performing, we no longer finished at midnight, we started at midnight. I became physically fatigued. Walking up the stairs to teach my class on the first floor was getting ridiculously difficult, but I kept pushing myself because I kept thinking, 'Why stop now?'

I remember looking in the mirror after getting up for a Sunday morning class, and I was a very pale shade of grey. I was fulfilling my childhood dream and living the life of a weekend rock star, but I realised that it wasn't worth it. My enthusiasm towards the school had waned and student numbers had started to drop off. I realised that my mind was disorientated. My relationship was strained and I was on the verge of leaving the family because it wasn't working.

It was then that I went to India for the first time to study with B.K.S. Iyengar. There, totally removed from the everyday demands of work and relationship, I felt that I was myself again. I could see what I had allowed to happen. I had taken on too many responsibilities, driven by self-centred priorities, and had lost myself among them all. I re-evaluated everything and went back home with definite ideas about what I was going to change in my life. But no matter what I did, I was not satisfied with my relationship. I was very frustrated and angry with myself, which disturbed my mental and emotional state, and in turn affected my teaching and practice. I pulled out all stops to re-establish my relationship, but finally, having exhausted every avenue, I decided the only option was to leave the family.

I fought with the idea of leaving my wife as a single mother and walking away from my children. Considering that I didn't have a father in my own childhood, it was a hard reality to confront. I resolved to leave because of the disturbed state I was in. I felt I was not fit to be a father, a husband or a teacher, because I was erupting inside with anger and rage. I decided that however drastic the measure, I had to change.

In that moment of extreme desperation, I remembered God—the universal life-giving energy—and I pleaded. 'I have exhausted every avenue. If there is something that I haven't thought of, give me a sign and show me how I can reconcile this relationship and restore peace within myself. I am about to take desperate measures and walk out.'

The answer resonated inside me.

'Your actions are not sincere. You think you want to heal your relationship, but in your heart, what is it that you really want?'

I had been behaving in a way that would get me out of trouble, but I wasn't being completely sincere. I was trying to fix my relationship with a 'Band-Aid'. My actions were mechanical, external gestures to appease my wife rather than to sincerely bring about change.

To explain how I felt, imagine that I am smiling, shaking your hand and saying, 'How are you? Pleased to meet you,' while in my mind, I am thinking how I can't stand you. There was an inconsistency between what I was feeling inside and how I was acting on the outside. I was trying to be a loving father to my sons but the truth was, I was too disturbed inside to sincerely care. Ironically, the same hypocrisy I had witnessed in the Italian boarding school that had made me anti-religious was now showing up in my own behaviour. I realised that I couldn't continue to live like this. I had to reconcile my attitude and actions. My obstacle was obsessiveness, motivated by the ego and fuelled by the emotions. The mind is attached to outcomes and expectations, whereas the heart is free from those conditions. I was missing the heart factor, which allows the expression of unconditional love.

To change my attitude, I remembered back to the start of my *asana* practice and how I was totally obsessed with the backbends, but had neglected the forward bends. My wife and children were my forward bends. I had been going with my likes and ignoring my dislikes and remained bound to the habitual conditioning of the mind. In the long run, it was this that caused great pain.

Now, sincerity of intention allowed me to detach from my conditions. My resistance fell away and enthusiasm returned for my family as it had for the forward bends.

The core of yoga is to transcend identifying with your conditions. Instead of being concerned with your like or dislike of a pose, remain focused on your intention behind your doing it and use that to measure the quality of your actions. Looking at Margaret and me today, you would never guess the trauma and pain we both suffered. I can't imagine not having this relationship in my life, and I can't imagine having this type of relationship with anybody else. We have a higher purpose and goal that keeps us together. Even when our conflicting personalities cause friction, we always sort it out, because our minds have become one in our spiritual endeavour.

My father died when I was ten years old. I think that had a great deal to do with my asking questions about life at an early age. I never resented that he'd been taken away because I felt that it was very much a part of who I was, and I was accepting of that. What it created, though, was a very strong urge to find out more about *who* I was. For that reason, in recent years I stripped back to the bone every aspect of my life, so as to look at who I really am and understand what motivates me.

Several years ago I moved with my wife and family to live in anonymity in northern New South Wales. In Melbourne, students put me on a pedestal. I stepped away from being 'Glenn Ceresoli, director of the Action School of Yoga'. I stood aside from my ambitions to teach around the world, and all the ego trappings that went with those ambitions. I stripped back everything, right down to what I ate: no sugar, coffee, ice cream. I stopped relying on anything that stimulated an image of myself that wasn't real. All of a sudden I found myself walking down the street in a very different manner.

It might sound like a mid-life crisis, but I call it the credit card syndrome. When you use a credit card, you are spending money you only *think* you have. It is a false perception. Similarly, a sugar hit makes you feel like you have energy when you don't. It is also possible to get false ideas about yourself, what you are doing and why you do it. I recognised this within myself and it became important to me to find the source of my motivation in teaching yoga. I believe that I have now reached a point where I can see more clearly the intention behind my thoughts, words and actions. Because of that clarity of intention the outer world can't seduce me so much anymore. I act with less ego and more heart.

Yoga has been a journey from the physical level, using the mental levels to finally arrive at and recognise the heart. Unlike the mind, the heart doesn't act from expectation of a particular outcome. The heart depends only upon the experience of its own expression, which is unconditional love.

Our culture is obsessed with 'doing'. As I have a lot of energy, enthusiasm and ambition, I was very good at 'doing'. But wh you're only *doing* something, you have a heavy expectation on the outcome of your efforts. You could call your effort an expense. The greater the expense, the more you expect a payback. If, however, you're doing something from the *being* aspect, you do it because it is an expression of the heart, and the expression becomes payment in itself. Our obsession with *doing* has become so great that we no longer give attention to *being*. To compensate for a lack of contentment, we try to do more and acquire more, but we keep looking outside of ourselves and contentment eludes us. There is little reflection upon our inner state. I prompt my inner process by asking myself what it is I am experiencing during my interactions with the outer world.

To honestly know what motivates your every action requires a very fine understanding of where your awareness is placed. It is an orientation of consciousness, and this is where yoga practices become the compass that always points north. Should I wish to travel east, west or south, I know my bearings and I don't get lost. I believe that we are divine beings having an earthly experience, and that we have been so lured and seduced by the sensory world that we have forgotten that we are spiritual beings. Our society is not like that of the past where the yogis used to withdraw into caves and isolate themselves from the outer world. Those yogis may have achieved great heights and states of consciousness, but they hadn't learnt how to deal with the world—they'd learnt how to deal without the world. In modern times it's more appropriate for us to be able to do both, to be equally aware inwardly and outwardly. Not to hide from the outer world, nor to ignore the inner world. Both must be achieved.

I have learnt that the severest setback in my life also allowed for the biggest revelations. What appeared to be a major obstacle was, in fact, a blessing because it led to greater understanding. When I was on the verge of walking out on my wife and children was when I learnt my biggest lesson about acting with sincerity, from the heart. Life no longer means making right or wrong actions, but simply complying with the consciousness of the heart. By transcending the mind's habitual conditions, you can live from the heart.

As a result of everything that happened in my life, my teaching has changed drastically from *how* to do yoga to *why* to do it. What are you aware of while you are doing your *asana* practice? What do you learn about yourself while attempting the poses?

Do yoga for the experience, don't just do it for the outcome of physical flexibility. You may think that by doing a certain pose you will stretch your hamstrings, and therefore gain greater flexibility, but as you are going through the process, look at what you experience. When you are intent on the experience of the action, the process effectively allows detachment from whatever results may or may not come. This helps bypass the mind's attachment to a payback for your output. This is what I have learnt, and this has been the pinnacle of my journey.

I am able to perceive my own life in greater depth, and have a greater ability to determine a student's stage of development because I have been there myself. I can ask myself, how did I get from where that person is to where I am now? Fifteen years ago, I would have been very pedantic about the exactness of alignment but now I see attitude and approach as the means to inner alignment.

The primary theme of my teaching is to present essential elements of yoga. Attitude and approach are key factors that free you from your habitual conditions and enable you to reach the core of your being. It is like taking the wrapping off a present to reach the gift. Yoga teaches how to unwrap the present with the least disturbance to what is inside. When someone first starts yoga, their attitude and approach are dictated by habitual conditions, their constitution and past experiences. For example, they might be short-tempered and fiery, or understanding and tolerant. Perhaps they were traumatised in childhood or maybe mollycoddled. Factors like this colour our approach to life, and therefore our approach to *asana* on the mat. The practice of yoga reveals to us our 'survival mode' nature and tries to raise our awareness from the level of survival to the higher aspects of our being. When I teach, I hope that people will contact that aspect of their Self [eternal, constant being] that will allow them to find the path—right, wrong or indifferent as it appears to the outside world—that is most appropriate to their journey.

As we retrain the body out of its tight and restricted conditions, the mind follows suit, and the ability to act deliberately and consciously replaces unconscious, reflex habits. Teaching yoga requires being as clear an instrument as possible so that what comes through is the yoga and not your own conditions. A teacher must endeavour to be as pure a vehicle as possible. Being a yoga teacher also means living for inspiration. Just as a musician lives to allow the music to come through, as a channel of expression, a yogi lives for the same thing: to explore and discover a new expression of movement and energy which brings them fully to life.

When I moved away from Melbourne, my colleagues told me that it was financial suicide. They thought I had a screw loose. People felt I was at the peak of my career and that I was stepping away from it. They couldn't understand my actions, but I knew that in the end it wouldn't matter how great a yoga teacher I became or how successful the school became or how much money I made. None of it mattered if I couldn't be true to myself and walk into my own home and feel the sanctity of love in my family.

Hatha yoga is union with God, whether you call that the cosmic force, higher intelligence, higher Self or love. There are many words used to describe the Absolute, but they are all inadequate. If your intention is to make that connection, then that's what you will gain from yoga. That is its ultimate purpose and essence. Yoga is a pathway to the ultimate. It reorientates and expands your perception from the outer to the inner world. It is like a street directory that can show you where you are and the potential of where you want to go. Yoga has taken me from living with a shallow intention, steeped in ignorance, to experiencing a depth of being and understanding because that is its function.

I can't imagine where I'd be without yoga. Undoubtedly I would have achieved a height in whatever field I chose simply because that's my make up. Whether it would have given me the same contentment, the same depth of understanding, the same fulfilment, I doubt very much. I would not have achieved the same degree of internal peace and satisfaction. I can honestly say I am content with my life. If you ask me, 'Do you feel content? Are you grateful? Do you feel satisfied internally for what you experience in your life?' My answer is YES!

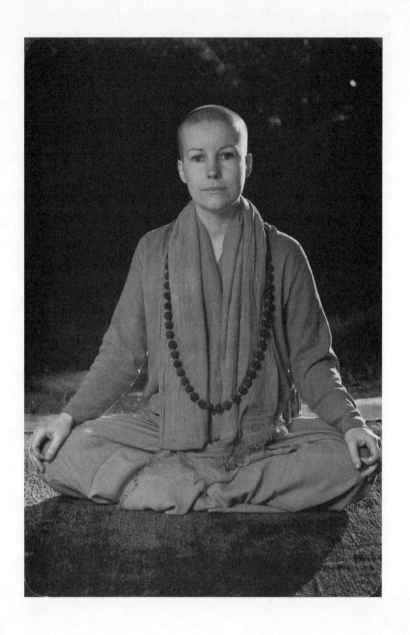

# 4

# CULTIVATING AWARENESS THROUGH A TRADITIONAL YOGA TRAINING

## *Muktanand Meannjin*

*As human beings, our greatness lies not so much in being able to remake the world . . . as in being able to remake ourselves.*

Mahatma Gandhi

*In the early seventies a psychology student with a keen interest in philosophy and yoga is* en route *to Europe. Her journey breaks in India where, to deepen her meditation practice, she plans a brief visit to the Bihar School of Yoga. What she does not know is that this place, its community and the person at its centre will transform her at the deepest level. The planned six-week stopover stretches into twelve years of intense inner study, and her voyage to Europe instead becomes a voyage into the essence of her being.*

*Although initially sceptical about the rigours of ashram life and ambivalent towards the notion of the 'guru', Muktanand Meannjin (as she became known) is attracted to the brightness of community life and, a day at a time, she decides to stay longer. After a year and careful consideration she takes* sannyas, *committing herself to the spiritual path. Eventually she leaves the ashram, though not by choice. Her guru, Swami Satyananda—the head of the ashram he founded in 1963 to impart traditional yogic training to all nationalities— requested that she establish a yoga ashram in his name in South India.*

*In 1986, twelve years after leaving for her European vacation, Muktanand comes home. She returns to the same lover she left behind, to the familiar world in which she grew up, and to resume her study of psychology, earning a Masters of Letters with the thesis, 'The Self: East and West'. But she is not the same person she was when she left. She is skinnier, she wears robes, her head is shaved and she goes by a different name. But those differences are superficial. The real change is beneath. She knows herself more clearly now.*

*To her delight she sees that yoga is offered everywhere! To her dismay she notices that there is little mention in these classes of the traditional practices and philosophy in which she was trained. In her own gentle way she sets about correcting the misconception that yoga means the practice of physical postures (asana) and that meditation is something only Buddhists do.*

*Muktanand has been a pioneer in restoring silent meditation retreats to their proper place in Australian yoga, and, at the invitation of Zen Master and Vipassana teacher Subhana Barzaghi, restoring yoga to its proper place in Buddhist retreats.*

*What follows is a frank disclosure of the intensity of the traditional training she received in the ashram. Muktanand explains why a traditional approach to yoga and meditation is important if yoga is to remain a practice of transformation in the west, as it has always been in the east.*

# SOMETHING MORE

When I look to my student days before I left for India, it is clear to me that, although young and naive, I was already searching. When you have embarked on an inner search and you come across something that answers a longing, your own inner light recognises it. Yoga was like that for me.

When I first encountered yoga it was 1969, a time of social foment—living in communes, protests against the Vietnam War, a resurgence of feminism, experiments with psychedelics and marijuana, and exploration of eastern mysticism. I was young and into everything but studying! In my spare time I did a lot of reading of philosophy and when I saw that yoga was offered at the university gym, I signed up. All I can recall of the class was a stern man sitting on a dais doing a difficult spinal twist that, looking back, I would never consider for beginners! There was no mention of philosophy. I didn't go back. Nevertheless, there must have been an internal recognition because I didn't dismiss yoga for good.

A few years later I left Sydney to join my lover, Kundan,

who had secured a lecturing job in Toowoomba, a small town in rural Queensland. There, I decided I would try yoga again. This time I loved it. Despite never being a physical person— I hated team sports and never liked exercise—I loved doing the postures. One day I remember going home after a very focused *pranayama* [breathing techniques] practice and announcing to Kundan that I was not going to smoke dope anymore. 'I can have the same sort of experiences through my yoga practice,' I told him, 'and it feels better this way.'

I could already feel a shift in consciousness taking place. Time slowed down, I could feel my awareness expanding, and my perception of life was altering. In those days, my practice wasn't all that deadly serious. It was more about feeling good than it was about self-exploration.

When I started working, I kept up a daily practice. I would walk to work—which was just a way of making money so that one day I could travel to London—and then come home in the afternoon and do about an hour and a half of yoga before dinner. Over about a two-year period, I began to get up earlier and earlier, around five o'clock in the morning in summer, to have enough time to read a passage from the *Bhagavad Gita* [a traditional yoga text] and contemplate it as I prepared for work.

Over time I found that the practices started taking me deeper and further along the path and I started looking for more. One of my teachers in Toowoomba happened to be a student of Swami Satyananda, and was trained to teach *mudra* [a physical gesture that affects the body's energy flow], *bandha* [a muscular contraction that alters the body's energy flow] and *pranayama* in the traditional style. I felt very inspired by her teaching and she felt very connected to Swamiji; eventually that was what would set me on the trail to meet Swami Satyananda. (Swami means one who has cultivated mastery over themselves; '-ji' denotes great affection and respect.)

In 1974, a senior disciple of Swami Satyananda, Swami Amritananda, was to visit Sydney. I made the trip down from Queensland and I told her that I was really interested in yoga and would like to go and live in an ashram. What I didn't tell her was that I assumed that if I did go she would be my teacher. At the time, because of the emergence of feminism, it was very important to me that my teacher be a woman. On that same trip I learnt that my yoga teacher's husband was leaving to visit the ashram in Bihar and, quite spontaneously, I decided to go along. I returned to Toowoomba, collected my money and passport, made travel arrangements, and within a week I was gone.

My plan was vague. I would spend a six-week stopover in India *en route* to Europe, during which time I would go to the ashram and learn what I could to deepen my yoga practice. I wasn't interested in staying in India; I knew nothing of its culture or its climate. In retrospect, I was astoundingly ignorant! I just went.

I had heard my teacher describe the Bihar ashram as being very hard, very primitive; consequently, I believed that a stay there would be a wonderful challenge. 'If I could survive this experience,' I thought, 'that would develop a great strength in me!' We arrived in India and went straight to the ashram. My first day there was either the day before or the day after my twenty-third birthday—I can't recall which now.

I remember how imposing the ashram compound felt when I first arrived. One of my strongest impressions was of the huge metal gates that were permanently locked and the twelve-foot high wall that encircled the grounds. But I also remember that once inside everything seemed very peaceful. The plot of land was only about one acre and it was bordered by a lagoon to one side, which was an offshoot of the Ganga [Ganges River], and a busy dirt road on the other. A railway line ran alongside, and three or four times a day trains would whistle by. In other words, the ashram wasn't situated in a particularly quiet place, but it was a very peaceful place. Nowadays there is a newer, much larger campus up on a hill—known as Ganga Darshan—and the old Bihar School of Yoga is now headquarters for the Sivananda Math (one of the organisation's charities).

I must have subconsciously held a romanticised vision that an ashram was a place of thatched-roof bungalows and flickering candlelight because what I found shocked me. The old Bihar School of Yoga was an austere brick and cement construction. The floors were polished cement, and fluorescent lights hung overhead. I was horrified!

The dormitory (men and women slept separately) was an empty hall furnished with nothing but beds called *chowkis*. A *chowki* was a low flat wooden base. Four sticks were arranged one at each corner, over which a mosquito net was draped at night. A futon mattress that was one inch thick—one inch!—went over the wooden base and we were each issued with a sheet and a thin pillow. Every morning when we got up we rolled up our bedding, stored it on a shelf and converted the bed into a table, and then began to work where we had just slept. We would sit on the floor with legs crossed because there were no chairs in the ashram—not one! Only the bare necessities were provided; the ashram was devoted to simple living.

An ashram literally means a place of intense inner work. *Shrama* means work or 'effort'. As is often the case in Sanskrit, the meaning is inverted. *A-shrama* means to turn away ordinary work in preference for inner work, from the material to the spiritual. Traditionally, an ashram is a hermitage where seekers live for spiritual training with a wise teacher.

A typical day in the ashram began with wake up at 3.30 a.m. or 4 a.m. You would get up and shower, only ever with cold water. This meant that in winter the water was bitterly cold, while in summer it was always lukewarm. Showering was regarded as part of the discipline. There was a great emphasis on cleanliness: keeping yourself clean, eating clean food and maintaining clean surroundings. The ashram was so clean that you could literally eat off the floor.

Between 4 and 6 a.m. you did your own practices and usually that meant meditation, maybe postures [*asana*] or *pranayama*. Breakfast was just after sunrise at 6 a.m. and it consisted of a cup of weak black tea with sugar. In winter you might also have a small handful of something to eat, like boiled chickpeas or unsweetened halva made with salt.

After breakfast, you went about your allocated work for the day. There was teaching to be done, as well as cleaning and cooking. One of the tasks the ashram undertook, and for which it is well known, was to write and produce books about yoga that were then distributed around the world. We participated in every aspect of the publishing of those books, from writing to typesetting to proofreading to binding and dispatching.

What made our work more interesting was that the equipment wasn't state-of-the-art, modern machinery. The printing press was fairly typical of one you might have found in the western world before any form of mechanisation was introduced. Words were spelt out one letter at a time and arranged onto what was called a 'stick'. A stick represented one line of text. You held the stick in your left hand, while your right hand fumbled through a box containing the alphabet in capitals, lower case, italics and so on. If the introductory page said: 'A book about yoga' you would pick up the letter 'A', then something that represented a space, then 'b', then 'o', and so on. To set one page of type in six hours was considered fairly fast. After the printing was complete we had to fold the pages and often bind the books ourselves.

At 10 a.m. we ate lunch, which was a full meal of rice, *chapatti*, vegetables and *dhal*. Half an hour later we went back to work. At 1.30 p.m. we had another cup of weak black tea. And then at 5 or 5.30 p.m., just before sunset, was dinner: rice, *dhal* and *chapatti*. The food was very simple, not at all spicy, and was varied according to the seasons.

After dinner we convened for *satsang* where Swamiji would sit and talk with us about yoga philosophy, or we would have *kirtan*, chanting and singing. Occasionally we would go back to work. By eight, we would go to our rooms and do our own practice, which was mainly meditation at that time of day. We went to sleep no later than nine.

The days were long. We often worked for twelve or fourteen hours and we didn't chat much. We were very focused on being mindful. In this way, everyday life provided total immersion in yoga. Even when on a break people had conversations over a cup of tea about an aspect of yoga philosophy or yoga practice. And yet although the immersion was intense, the atmosphere in the ashram wasn't solemn or heavy, it was very bright and enthusiastic.

There was an understanding among ashramites that if you found your way to the ashram, then you were meant to be there. What drew most people was their connection with the guru. What was unusual in my case was that I didn't feel an immediate connection with Swami Satyananda. I had no idea what a swami was or even what a guru was and I certainly wasn't looking for one! What I was primarily interested in was yoga and the idea of community—remember, this was the early seventies and there was a lot of social change happening. While I wasn't keen on the hippie-style, return-to-the-earth communities where the day was spent growing your own vegetables and weaving your own cloth, I *was* interested in the idea of community as opposed to nuclear family. I guess that is why I never entertained the idea of living in a cave; I wanted to live in a community with others. Because I also wanted to know more about yoga, living in an ashram seemed ideal.

## BE AWARE!

The Bihar School of Yoga was a Karma yoga ashram, meaning that the primary practice was working with awareness. We did all kinds of yoga practices in the ashram—cleansing practices, postures, breathing practices, chanting, meditation—but the central focus was Karma yoga, meditation in action, and it cultivated awareness in everyday life.

There was no motto in the ashram as such, but if there had been it would have been 'be aware'. There were constant reminders to remain vigilant of our thoughts and actions at all times, even in innocuous ways. For example, outside the complex of rooms where Swamiji lived there was a passageway that led to the printing press. Because the buildings had been constructed at different times not all the doorways were the same height and the doorway at the end of this passageway was particularly low. For a small person like me this posed no problem, but for a medium to tall person this was potentially hazardous. Each time someone walked under this doorway they would have to remember to lower their head, or else bang it. So you see, constant awareness was crucial even in small ways!

The swamis carried out most of the work of the ashram. If you were a visiting student, there were no set tasks for you to do unless you asked. When I first arrived and was just visiting, I didn't want to sit around so I went to Swamiji and said I would like to make a contribution. He sent me to the printing press to work with an American, Swami Bhaktanand. Bhaktanand was on a vow of silence, so instead of speaking to me he would write notes. The first task he gave me was to prepare a glossary for the book called *Meditations from the Tantras*, which is a compendium of different meditation practices that are taught as part of the Satyananda tradition. I did this willingly. Next Bhaktanand wrote me a note asking, 'Can you type?' Shocked, I replied definitively: 'No!' Typing was a skill I had purposely not learnt because I never wanted to be a secretary to anyone. Bhaktanand wrote back baffled, 'Why not?' Before I knew it he had sat me down on the bare cement floor at one of these low tables that had been someone's bed the night before, put a typewriter in front of me and gave me a bundle of transcribing to do. I was infuriated!

I complied, and then I drifted off and befriended a much older woman, Swami Shantanand, who became a mentor to me and who I grew to love very much. I asked her any questions that arose for me and I worked with her for some time. When Swamiji found out that I had drifted off, he put me back to work in the press. There I was given some typesetting to do, which I found excruciatingly boring. I literally wept, day after day, as I sat there. I wept as I painstakingly placed each letter on the 'stick' and wondered what I was doing there. I wept with frustration and I wept with boredom.

Every now and then I reminded myself that I had come to learn yoga and not how to type, and so I went to Swamiji to tell him that it was time for me to leave. One time he replied, 'Why don't you go back to Australia and be a yoga teacher?' I was stunned. I responded, 'How can I go back to Australia to teach what I don't know anything about? I haven't had a chance to learn anything while I have been here!'

A course in *kundalini kriyas* [advanced bodily positions and energetic gestures that powerfully move the practitioner into a deeper state of consciousness] was soon to begin—he suggested I do it and the course gave me a real boost. In the coming years, whenever I wanted to leave, Swamiji would give me something to keep me there, like the job of creating a Sanskrit dictionary that involved me reading all the texts on Tantra written by Sir John Woodroffe, a British judge of the High Court of Calcutta who wrote extensively on Indian philosophy and spirituality in the 1920s under the *nom de plume*, Arthur Avalon. Work like this appealed to my intellectual side very much.

Even though I stayed at the ashram, I still wasn't convinced that I would become a swami. What I found very difficult to abide by was the discipline. The first time I had to get up at 4 a.m. I squealed in protest and demanded to know what was going on. 'The sun hasn't even risen! Why are you doing this to me?' I was told that I had to get up and help clean, so I did. I got up, I cleaned, then I went straight back to bed! Nobody could believe I did this but, you see, nobody had explained the reason behind the tradition of getting up at 4 a.m. You learnt by osmosis. I learnt later that yogis rise 'two hours before sunrise' because this is the time of day that we are most psychically receptive and it is a very potent time to meditate.

## LIKE IN MIND, KINDRED IN SPIRIT

Part of Swami Satyananda's undertaking was 'To take yoga from door to door and shore to shore . . .' I suppose it was what you would call his 'mission statement', but it was more an encapsulation of his vision for yoga. As part of that, Swamiji attracted and trained students from all over the world. People take it for granted now that anyone who was interested in learning more about yoga could do so, but at the time this was very special.

To find a very traditional ashram that would accept western-ers was unusual—most traditional lineages don't. The idea, especially, of teaching the more esoteric aspects of yoga to westerners was extremely rare. But the other very unusual factor, at the time, was that Swami Satyananda welcomed women. Even organisations that would teach women the yoga practices wouldn't allow them to take *sannyas* [initiation to become a yogic monk] or to reside in the ashram for training. Swami Satyananda did. First he accepted Indian women as *sannyasins* [yogic equivalent of monk], then he accepted western women, and that was a very radical thing to do. It was viewed as breaking tradition and he was criticised for it. Nowadays it is much more acceptable to teach women and western women.

Swami Satyananda felt that women had a lot of spiritual potential and that they should not be denied the opportunity to develop that potential. In the ashram, he put women in leadership roles and gave them responsibility. Even so, life in the ashram was mostly gender neutral, right down to our names. This was partly a reflection of the nature of the Self, which transcends gender, but it was also a reflection of his genuine encouragement of people—male or female—according to the potential that he saw in them and their dedication to the path.

To the same degree that the Bihar School of Yoga was considered radical for being inclusive of women and westerners, it was also seen as traditional. Living by the traditional teachings was one of the strengths of the ashram.

It frequently occurred to me that on this one acre plot of land we had a gathering of women and men who had almost nothing in common except for a profound interest in yoga and commitment to working with this particular teacher. We were all dedicated to studying, growing and learning harmoniously, but at the same time, the range of opinions, perspectives and personalities among us was exceptionally wide. Adding to the often dynamic mix of energies was the fact that most of us were in our twenties or early thirties.

To understand the nature of the ashram, I feel that a distinction needs to be made between a commune and a spiritual community. A commune is a place where people have a lot of ideas in common, and a big emphasis is placed on interrelationship between the members. In the ashram we were a spiritual community where the emphasis was not so much on relationships with each other as on the path and with the teacher. If you were to liken an ashram to another form of spiritual community, it would be most similar to a monastery.

Being a part of such a community was a byproduct of the whole process, and while it presented its own challenges, it also provided a very strong sense of support and deep bonding. To this day, the people I trained with are like family—on one level, they are more like family than blood family. And even though we've done diverse things since leaving the ashram, and all of those differences in politics, opinions and personal style have reasserted themselves, whenever we meet there is an unconditional acceptance and a deep affection between us. The supportive connection is very deep.

Despite the fact that we lived in a community, there was a great inwardness of focus. We lived this paradox of personal inward focus and outward connectedness. In my reading I came across a passage by Antoine de St Exupery in *Wind, Sand and Stars* that expresses this beautifully: 'No one can draw a free breath who does not share with others a common and disinterested ideal. Life has taught us that love does not consist in gazing at each other but in looking outward in the same direction. There is no comradeship except through union in the same high effort.'

## MAKING A CONSCIOUS COMMITMENT

My planned six-week stay passed quickly but it was nearly a year before I decided that I would take *sannyas*. I was already a part of the community, I had already shaved my head, and for all intents and purposes, I was already living the life of a *sannyasin*. But this was a decision that I weighed up seriously.

People automatically expected that I would take *sannyas* because there was this understanding that if you really wanted to go further in yoga, if you really wanted to pursue it to the full extent, you would take this initiation and become a *swami*

(swami is the title given to a *sannyasin*). It was understood that you could also pursue this path as a householder [a married man or woman with worldly duties], but this was considered to be less intense and the path less sure. If you were really committed, you would take initiation into *sannyas*.

I was initiated along with three other swamis at *Guru Poornima* in July 1975. *Guru Poornima* is a big festival that occurs on the mid-summer full moon, said to be the brightest light of the year. Whether you are a householder or a *sannyasin*, this is a time of respect and gratitude for your guru and all that they have given you, and a time to recommit to your practices. People in India travel long distances to visit their teacher and to make an offering to their teacher's work. It is a big day on the yoga calendar and an auspicious day. Initiations are always conducted at these spiritually pivotal times.

My initiation didn't involve the taking of vows. Swami Satyananda always said that taking a vow was an invitation to break it. Regardless of formal vows, we did live celibacy, poverty and obedience—these were the realities of our life. We lived celibacy in that sexual relationships in the ashram were strongly discouraged. We lived poverty in that we didn't even own the clothes we wore. (Our ochre robes—the dhoti, long sleeve Nehru shirt, and upper dhoti or shawl—were all given to us.) And, of course, we lived obedience to our teacher and the way of life in the ashram. Doing what you were told to do was an essential discipline in ashram life.

The initiation ceremony took place around a fire. Beforehand our heads were cleanly shaven, save one lock of hair that the guru would later shave. We then bathed completely and put on our new robes. We were also given a *rudrakshamala*, a string of 108 prayer beads made of seeds, *rudraksha*, that are said to be the 'eye of Shiva'. We went to the fire ceremony where there was a lot of chanting.

The fire ceremony was a symbolic baptism by fire. In it, you burnt up all your existing attachments and your previous ways of self-identification. For instance, if you were an Indian man who wore a thread across one shoulder to denote the Brahmin caste, then you put that into the fire because you renounced caste. A crucifix, photographs, anything that represented family or class or caste or who you thought you were, any means of social definition, as opposed to spiritual definition, also went into the fire. Swamiji then completed the head shave and threw the remnants of our hair into the fire, symbolising the cutting off of all our past ways of looking at life and hence everything that bound us to a limited self.

We were also given a yoga name to represent our inner essence. In Indian culture, the name your parents give you is a strong indicator of where you fit into society. From your name people can tell your caste, whether your family worshipped Shiva or Vishnu or Shakti, and other things like this. So part of the renunciation included setting aside your old name, the name of your limited social self, and taking on a name that represented a part of yourself of which you were unaware or which needed development. Your name became a kind of *mantra*, a reminder of your potential.

My full name was Swami Muktananda Saraswati. *Mukta* means 'free from attachment' or 'free from spiritual ignorance'. Someone who is *mukta* is someone who recognises they are not bound. *Ananda* means 'bliss', and it is a common ending for a swami's name. Saraswati is the name of my lineage. In India, there are ten orders of *sannyasins*, and the Saraswati order is a Karma yoga order to which my teacher, Swami

Satyananda, belongs. Carrying on this name is an important representation of continuing the line of inspiration from teacher to student unbroken.

To accept a name that someone else imposes upon you in adulthood is an interesting exercise and I had a very strong reaction to it that partly stemmed back to my feminist beliefs. When I left Australia, it was amidst the budding feminist movement of the early seventies, but even before that I had a strong feminist spirit. My mother had brought me up to believe that women are just as good as men and should be able to do jobs like men, not marry too young, and so on.

When I left Australia I was young and still learning to define myself as separate from my family, which included a very domineering father figure, and I was very sensitive about feminist issues, or 'women's lib' as it was known then. Any action or attitude that looked to me like it was relegating women into a traditional role, or limiting them in some way, I would speak out about, even to Swamiji.

Sometimes when I spoke out I was not as tactful as I could have been and people were often shocked at my boldness. So when I was told that my name was to be Muktanand, naturally I asked, 'What does it mean?' The reply came: 'It means liberated.' I thought it was some joke that they were having at my expense—about being a 'liberated woman'—and I was very upset.

Having a name given to you in this way becomes another means of spiritual practice. It prompts self-examination. How do I feel about this? Do I or don't I like it? What does it mean? How can I live up to it? Am I living up to it? In the same way that wearing robes and shaving your head are ways of removing all those masks and projections we use to define ourselves socially, our spiritual name permits a similar inner freedom.

When the masks are removed—who you thought you were, your idea of yourself as a public person—you have to face the discomfort of not having anything to hide behind, but after that there is a lot of freedom to be found.

I loved having my head shaved! In fact I loved it so much that in the months leading up to taking *sannyas*, Swamiji instructed me to stop shaving my head, which I found very difficult, even though I had arrived in the ashram with long hair. Nowadays a shaved head is seen as a fashion statement, but back then it wasn't. The barber would come in once a month and shave you to the scalp. That was confronting because there was no way to influence attractiveness, or how people perceived you—but it was also very beautiful, because a shaved head is very revealing of your whole face. After years of shaving my head, I didn't ever want to have hair again because I felt that it obscured people seeing into the real person.

On an energetic level, shaving your head helps to disperse the inner heat, or transforming energy, which you are generating through your practices, particularly when you are practising celibacy. This heat rushed out so quickly on the first day our heads were shaved that we had to wear something to cover the scalp. On a simpler level, shaving is hygienic, and this is practical when living in India.

Wearing the robes was also a discipline, but there was real freedom in knowing what you were going to wear each day. You didn't have to fuss about it and spend time thinking about what to put on! And even though our clothes were the same— we all wore the ochre robes—there was never uniformity in the way that we wore them. Everyone had his or her own way of tying a dhoti or wrapping a shawl.

Wearing the robes and shaving your head also removed

gender association. I remember visiting Bangalore, in the south of India, at a time when I was very thin, wearing these very concealing robes with a shaved head. A lot of people assumed I was a young boy, only I didn't realise this at first. I was staying with a host family in Bangalore and I wanted to have my head shaved, so they called a barber to the house. Later on, another swami visited that same town and also went to have his head shaved and the barber asked after the wellbeing of the little boy swami. It turned out that he was referring to me!

Another time, I was staying with a family and they invited people to come to their home and meet me. A man in his seventies arrived and he kept asking me, 'Aren't you young to be living this life?' I joked with him that I wasn't as young as I looked and he answered, 'But you are so young, you don't even have any hair on your face yet!' I suddenly realised he thought I was a boy. What this meant was that I felt very protected; I could move around freely without being harassed or feeling fearful.

Not everyone took kindly to seeing a westerner dressed in robes. One day, also in Bangalore, I had gone to town to buy food for the ashram and a man came up to me and started haranguing me about the significance of wearing robes in his country, and how dare I wear them! He was very angry. He thought I was dressing up like this to play with fashion. I tried to talk to him about Swami Satyananda, and also Swami Sivananda, who was Swamiji's guru and who is very well known in South India, and eventually he calmed down. Indians treat taking *sannyas* very seriously.

After I took *sannyas*, I didn't feel that much changed for me in practical terms. Before I took it, however, I agonised over the decision because it meant making a commitment not only to my inner life but also to an unusual and rigorous lifestyle. It also meant accepting what my guru allocated me to do, whether I liked it or not, as best for my spiritual growth.

## ACCELERATING ONE'S EVOLUTION

At the beginning of 1976 Swamiji decided that there would be intense *sannyasa* training. This was a rigorous residential training to be conducted over three years (1976–78) for newly initiated swamis and people who wanted to become swamis. People gathered from all over India and the world. The number of people living in the ashram swelled from around thirty to over sixty. Half came from around India, and there were equal numbers of men and women. This meant the ashram would be closed to outside visitors except during the summer holidays when devotees from different parts of India could visit. There were to be no tourists, no casual visitors coming and going, and people who lived in the ashram were not to go out.

The location of the ashram was such that the physical conditions were intense. Bihar School of Yoga is situated in the northeast of India, in the state of Bihar, an area that is inland from Calcutta and which lies between Patna and Gaya. This particular area has one of the highest variations in temperature anywhere in the world. In the winter it can be zero degrees at night, while in the summer it can soar to 48 degrees or above. During the monsoon the heat is further accentuated by a sweltering humidity.

When I first arrived, it was during the monsoon and I thought I was going to die from the heat. I could hardly breathe and yet all the Indians kept saying, 'This is so much cooler!' I would come to learn that it *was* much cooler than the summer! My first summer, I remember working on the verandah in the morning and getting up from where I was sitting to see, literally, a pool of sweat behind me. I can remember eating and eating and getting thinner and thinner. The heat was draining. So life wasn't just emotionally challenging, but physically challenging too.

Day-to-day life was also challenging, and intentionally so. There were not a lot of comforts in the ashram. In the winter it was a challenge to shower. Some days in the middle of winter, we would take a bucket, fill it with cold water in the morning, leave it in a sunny place until midday, and then have a shower later in the day when the sun had slightly warmed the water.

Another creature comfort we soon did without was cosy bedding. And sleep. We got by on only the minimum amount, an average of six hours a night. The food was very pure in the sense that it was simple, clean and strictly vegetarian—we ate no dairy products and rarely sweets. The lack of luxuries wasn't really a question of being made to feel uncomfortable—it was a question of exploring our limits, physically, and mentally, and then extending them.

In addition to our common work and study, Swamiji personalised a specific yoga program for each of us. Amazingly, he managed to do this for all sixty individuals in the ashram. He kept an eye on each of us. Perhaps every six months or so, Swamiji would give individual instruction for the practice of a meditation technique, *pranayama* or postures according to our individual concerns at the time, or whatever he recognised our need to be. Alongside these formal practices, our main practice was always to work with awareness. We were to work mindfully, to watch our reactions to events throughout the day, and to constantly observe our reactions to the conditions of the ashram.

And this happened in seemingly unintentional ways too—for instance, with regard to food.

Unlike wandering Buddhist monks, we weren't obliged to beg in the street for our meals, but like beggars we had to eat what we were given and the amount was usually spare. You might be able to ask for more, or less, but you couldn't say, 'I don't like this *dhal*, I want something else,' or, 'I'm tired of rice. Today I'll go out for pizza.' Instead, if you were displeased with dinner, you observed your reactions. There was no escaping the conditions of ashram life and that is what made the experience so intense. If things were disturbing for you, then you had to face them. And things did come up.

We had to learn to get along with everyone, one way or another. Again Swami Satyananda's influence came to bear. If there was somebody you didn't like, then, sure enough, you would be put to work alongside that person. Similarly, if you had a particularly close friend, then situations would be engineered to place you apart. You had to manage how you felt, and this became a form of practice.

Our roles in running the ashram were similarly designated to challenge us. The person in charge of the day-to-day running of the press was a well-known South American artist. Here was someone extremely talented at drawing and painting but with absolutely no management skills given the task of overseeing a printing press! What's more, she was a woman. Most of the workers in the press were male and they had to get used to the fact that they had a female boss. The situation was quite deliberately engineered by Swamiji, and was more radical at that time than it would be now.

One of the assumptions people make about living in an ashram is that it is full of love and light and there are no hard feelings. But when you are put in situations that confront you in fundamental ways, like not having hot water, one of the first emotions that comes up is anger. All of us went through stages of feeling angry, and it was a matter of finding a way of working through or transcending that anger. Because there was no escaping the situation—you couldn't just go out for a coffee or think, 'I have had it today! I'm going to watch TV!'— you had to find some insight into why you felt the way you did. Yet something unexpected and powerful also arose from this experience. Because everyone went through this, other ashramites recognised what was happening. We understood from our own experience that the anger arose out of the baggage we brought from our pasts. When we acted out our anger, we soon discovered that it hurt us more than it hurt others. Then we were able to experience the acceptance, even forgiveness, of the rest of the community—this was very powerful.

Everyone was working towards the same goal of exploring and embodying their essence. This included exploring the dark, shadow aspects of our personalities. Though usually quite painful, it enabled greater empathy and compassion for other people to develop. We learnt to look deeper than superficial personality.

That everybody shared the same ideals was very supportive. This cannot be underestimated; outside an ashram situation people have to struggle to establish a daily spiritual practice because the rest of the world doesn't necessarily value inner work.

So ashram life may sound austere, uncomfortable or challenging, but there was a purpose behind being put into such situations: to train us to go beyond our preferences. We cannot control everything in life. We can't cushion ourselves indefinitely and we cannot avoid suffering. At the very least, we are going to age and we are going to get sick at some time. If we don't know ourselves, we don't become the full person that we can be.

If conditions in life were always easy, then there would be no inner conflict to make us realise how limiting and restrictive our ingrained ideas and conditioned beliefs can be. Being confronted with a situation where we feel uncomfortable can be very useful in enhancing our awareness. For example, when somebody irritated me, I couldn't just avoid them, I had to look at myself instead. I had to examine my projections and ask myself, 'Why am I in this situation?' What I learnt about myself didn't necessarily translate into love for that person, but I found a way to rise above the irritation or dislike or whatever was the cause of the conflict. In this way, you ceased to be bound or limited by a particular issue.

Perhaps this sounds like a hard life, but one thing you have to remember is that our time in the ashram was only intended to be one part of our life. These conditions were not meant to last indefinitely. Our training was designed to establish a foundation. It was a time of personal exploration and inner strengthening, of gaining insights and self-knowledge. Swamiji referred to it as 'accelerating one's evolution'. It was like living in a pressure cooker.

Ultimately this sort of training was intended to help us gain insight into the relativity of personality. You realised that you didn't have to identify with being a particular kind of person. I might tend to be a particular kind of person, but it is good to be aware of that and not to regard it as fixed or absolute. Recognising this gives us an awareness that other people are also more than just their immediate, obvious personalities. Our training wasn't designed to eradicate our personalities, but to develop our ability to perceive the truth and totality of who we really are.

What I have been describing probably doesn't conform to most people's idea of what an ashram is and how it works. But, for me, ashram life was a very integrated experience. There weren't separate compartments marked: 'Yoga', 'Spiritual Development' and 'The Rest of Life'. There wasn't a split between spiritual life and working life. It was all integrated—and that is in keeping with the nature of yoga itself. If you wanted to sum up why we put ourselves through all this, well, the aim of yoga is to become a complete person, to become fully alive. To be fully alive we need flexibility of mind more than we need flexibility of body.

Swamiji was training yoga teachers but more than that he was training what he referred to as 'spiritual masters', people who were firmly established in the traditional practice. His idea was to produce people who were not just passing on techniques, but who could embody the teaching in their lives, and, in so doing, exemplify the teaching's depths.

## THE GURU KNOWS BEST

The relationship with the guru is complex and often hard for westerners to understand. It does not necessarily equate to a warm and fuzzy, Santa Claus-type of adoration. You are living with a reality: this person is a wise person, but a human being nonetheless. It is his or her job to be confronting in order for you to grow. When you are living closely with somebody who is revealing your strengths and your limitations, it is bound to create a complex relationship. That there is confrontation present makes it difficult to romanticise the guru relationship, which westerners often do. Nor does living with the guru automatically induce mindless devotion. Many westerners have an unreal expectation about what a teacher is able to do and so offer blind devotion, always touching the guru's feet (a very potent symbol in Indian culture). You just don't do this, and certainly Swamiji never required it!

The truth is that when I first arrived in the ashram I had no idea of what a guru really was. Because of that, my respect for Swamiji wasn't immediate, but something that grew. *Guru* literally means 'light in the dark'. A guru is therefore someone who can throw light on your darkness, the ignorance of your true nature. I remember telling someone that I wasn't looking for a guru, I just wanted to know more about yoga! I didn't want this intense teacher relationship; I didn't see that I needed it. In retrospect I am incredibly grateful for the experience of living in the ashram with Swamiji. If there was a downside—being his human foibles—the upside was that you got to witness how this person lived life on a day-to-day basis. Sometimes what you learnt was not so much technique but a prudent approach to the ordinary aspects of life. Swamiji set up situations that made a profound difference to who I am and to how I live my life. For that I feel immense respect and gratitude towards him.

The most obvious aspect of the guru–disciple relationship is learning to accept that there is somebody who knows what you need, and to trust in that. This is based on the notion that the guru knows more about the path than you do. Initially I had some difficulty with being told what to do, partly because I expected that what I needed to learn would be something I liked! Conflict arose when I had to do things that, to me, seemed irrational or against all common sense, not to mention emotion-ally confronting. A 'disciple' is one who follows the discipline, and learning obedience was an essential part of the discipline. Learning to obey the guru's instruction was a training-ground for learning to obey my own inner guidance. Like the guru, our own inner guidance doesn't always prompt us to do things that will be pleasant or easy, but if we ignore that inner prompting we miss out on something valuable.

It is widely acknowledged within the yogic tradition that the function of the physical outer guru is to awaken our own inner guru, which might also be called intuition. Before we can rely on this for guidance, we have to learn to distinguish between intuition and impulse. Our intuition will sometimes point us to things that are unpleasant or that we resist—it can direct us in ways that are hard to follow. Ultimately, practising obedience to an outer guru strengthened my relationship with my own inner guidance, and I came to see that as a tremendous gift.

What was truly remarkable was that what Swamiji did for me, he did for all his students. He kept a finger firmly on the pulse of ashram life, noting people's likes and dislikes and orchestrating situations that would encourage growth. These situations allowed us to experiment with ourselves. Sometimes there would not be enough food because he would have instructed the kitchen to make less. I am a small person, so fortunately I didn't need much food, but some of the ashramites were really big, tall men and some of them may have gone hungry more than once. Such situations created quite a furore, but you had to use your training to see that the problem only existed if you assumed the situation would continue forever. If you could look at it as something that was happening now and would pass, then you could observe your reactions instead.

It wasn't designed to be punitive. The experiment wasn't to see who could manage on less food, but to witness what happens when the things you depend on change.

Sleep is another aspect of everyday life that yogis traditionally experiment with. One way that people on the Tantric path confront fear of death is to meditate in the graveyard, especially at night. The ashram wasn't very far from the burning *ghats*, but Swamiji never encouraged us to go there. Instead, sometimes we would be woken at 1 or 2 a.m. and told to go to work in the press. One particular winter Swamiji had some of us working in the press around the clock. We worked through the night, but we couldn't go to sleep during the day when the rest of the ashram was up and about—we had to continue our work.

I vividly recall one three-month period over the winter of 1976 when I averaged two hours sleep per night. It was a totally non-traditional take on the traditional practice of sitting up and meditating through the night. It had a similar effect by allowing me to watch how sleep, or lack of sleep, affected my mood, my cycles of energy throughout the day, the clarity of my concentration, and how I interacted with people under those circumstances.

There was a lot to be learnt. I was in my twenties, living a life that promoted energy, and I remember thinking how much could be accomplished if I didn't have to sleep! I enjoyed not having to sleep and I learnt to work my way through the fuzzy times. Just when I got accustomed to it, Swamiji brought the experiment to a halt. Just when I learnt to embrace it and vowed never to sleep again he said, 'Okay, lights out!' The practice then became about watching how I responded to that change. In these ways, Swamiji oversaw our growth.

Just as Swamiji deliberately created this hothouse atmosphere, encouraging us to extend our boundaries, there were also times when he saw that we had gone far enough and he would declare a holiday. Here was a kind of risk, if you like, of reverse addiction. Too much food: you become addicted to food. Too little food: you become addicted to lack of food and the high that comes from that. The same happened with sleep. To become addicted to sleeping was to become slothful and lazy, and yogis are totally against that. But it was equally undesirable to become addicted to not sleeping. There should be no addictions. Swamiji would ensure that we didn't become extreme. There should be wisdom in what you are doing and a freedom from binding the self in any way.

Even though all of this sounds very challenging, perhaps severe, I should stress again that the atmosphere in the ashram was very bright and positive. There wasn't a sombre tone. There was laughing and joking and a feeling of lightness. This was largely due to our practice of Karma yoga. When we bring all our awareness to whatever we are doing, we slip through the barrier of thought and mind into essence, and this generates wellbeing, lightness and joy.

Another thing that I believe kept the atmosphere of the ashram light was the practice of celibacy within a mixed sex group. Swamiji was a Tantrik (he had trained under two Tantric gurus before he went to Swami Sivananda) and he recognised the benefits of mixing male and female energies. He thought the customary single sex ashrams were unnatural and unhealthy, and didn't help the spiritual process. We practised restraint, while avoiding the suppression of sexual energy.

Sexual relationships were actively discouraged—men and women slept separately, and there were more than one set of locked gates between them—but again, that wasn't necessarily intended for life. Limitations on food, asceticism, the practices of *mudras* and *bandhas*: all these helped to manage and redirect sexual energy and provide fuel for our meditation practices instead. On top of that, our days were long and physically strenuous, spent hauling buckets of water, cleaning and working with the heavy machinery in the press. Despite the celibacy, sexual energy wasn't being suppressed as such—it was just expressing itself differently. The dynamic between men and women, and the interplay between male and female energy, was present and very valuable and probably contributed to some of the lightness and joy in the ashram.

Swamiji gave us one-on-one instruction for formal practice, and he orchestrated situations for group learning, but there was one other dimension to his teaching that is hard to articulate, let alone to explain. This was a kind of psychic transmission, non-verbal instruction or energy transfer that took place. Swamiji's instructions still continue in my life, coming through dreams in which he or other teachers appear, as a form of blessing or initiation or formal instruction. It is hard to explain but it is very real.

Even though I left the ashram in 1985, the understanding of Swamiji's teaching is still revealing itself to me. There were times when Swamiji did or said things I didn't agree with, or didn't approve of, or couldn't understand the rationale for, but many years later, when I found myself in a similar situation, I would recall his behaviour and suddenly I understood. It was as if the seeds were planted while in the ashram, but the comprehension and knowledge continues to unfold.

A good *guru-chela* [teacher–student] relationship is one of inspiration not of dependence. You would find that those of us who underwent Swamiji's training and who are now teaching yoga are teaching from the strength of a shared lineage and from a common body of techniques developed by Swami Satyananda and furthered by Swami Niranjan [Swami Satyananda's successor], but we are each doing this with our own unique flavour. The relationship with the guru is not supposed to eradicate personality or turn you into a duplicate of your teacher. It is intended that you will incorporate the wisdom and insight of your guru's teachings into your own nature, so that you can become more truly who you are.

It is my experience, and that of many others, that we reach a certain point where we need to reclaim our inner guru and to do so might involve conflict with our outer guru. Often a situation will arise where you must choose between the guru's advice and your own deep inner guidance. This won't happen in the early stages of your practice, but only after you have reached a certain level of maturity. The point is that you are able to leave the guru's company and still stay steadfast on the path. In my case it took the form of a conscious decision, which Swamiji respected.

## TEACHING YOGA TO INDIANS

I spent nearly five years in my guru's ashram in Bihar and for several of those I didn't leave the compound, neither to go to the markets (which a swami did to bring back food for everyone) nor to the Ganga to swim or to bathe (which we always did as a group and which was considered a special privilege). In time Swamiji would send me from Bihar in the northeast to Bangalore in the south where I would establish a new ashram in his name.

I spent most of my last year under Swamiji's instruction

meditating in a cave on the ashram grounds. When the ashram was first constructed, and occasionally afterwards, Swami Satyananda lived in this cave and used it for his own practices. No one had been invited to use it since. Swamiji asked me to use that space and gave me a particular meditation practice to do. He asked me to keep silent, not to interact with anyone, and to see if I could write a book on *samadhi* [union with universal consciousness], for which I prepared (though did not finish) by making an intense study of Patanjali's *Yoga Sutras*.

Each day I had set periods of meditation, one in the early morning, another in the middle of the day, and again in the late afternoon. I lived in strict isolation. No one was to come to the cave and I was not to interact with anyone. The intensity of the practice was challenging but at the time I was ready for it. I took it very seriously and, in some ways, I loved it.

Those ten months of silence and meditation opened my eyes to the benefits of the *mouna*, or noble silence. It conserves energy, maintains your connection with the inner world undisturbed by conversation, and it throws your thoughts into relief. When you are not speaking, you become aware of how often you would have voiced a thought. You begin to see more clearly the pattern of your thoughts and even the impulses that lead you to communicate, or not to communicate. Silence is very self-revealing and nourishing.

So I spent the last ten months in the ashram like this, in silence, in isolation and in meditation. My subsequent teaching of meditation is rooted deeply in that experience.

I was not a teacher at that time, but afterwards Swami Satyananda asked me to start teaching. Teaching was seen as a combination of privilege and natural inclination. In order to teach, you had to have passed through an inner purification and inner strengthening and to have reached a place where you can be a teacher without attaching a lot of ego to it. You can be a channel for the teachings without being 'The Teacher'.

For most of us having to teach was seen as a bit of a bother—it was one more thing that we had to fit into our routine. On the other hand, there was a sense that something more was being asked of you. Those of us who had started teaching also recognised that it helped facilitate our own practice. One of the best ways to learn something is to teach it. You have to find ways to integrate it and to understand the process well enough to be able to articulate it clearly to another person. We used to talk about how teaching prevented 'spiritual constipation'; if you learnt and learnt and learnt and never passed it on, it somehow blocked your own progress.

Towards the end of my time in the cave, some people from South India approached Swamiji to request that a female swami be sent to set up women-only classes in Bangalore. Because they had read the book I had written in 1977, *Nawa Yogini Tantra* (Yoga for Women) they were particularly interested in having me teach them and so Swamiji sent me to South India. For me, the timing seemed abrupt. I came out of solitary practice in the cave and straight into a very public teaching role. And so this became another kind of training for me.

I had been in Bangalore for about six months when Swamiji visited and the local people told him that they wanted to establish an ashram and asked if I could stay permanently. Swamiji agreed and I remained in Bangalore for a further seven years. The ashram was called *Atma Darshan Yogashram*, which means 'Vision of the True Self'. We taught yoga practices in the Satyananda tradition and conducted a lot of yoga therapy training. It was unusual for a westerner to be in a position of teaching yoga and meditation to Indians, but for the most part people were very receptive and really appreciative of the Satyananda approach to the teachings.

It was nothing for me to have a class of sixty women, sometimes one hundred at a time, with just one or two students to help me. It was a huge challenge for a teacher and it demanded an enormous simplification of language. In India there are fourteen major languages. In Bangalore alone there are three—Kannada, Tamil and Telegu—and a lot of the women attending the classes barely understood English. It was a very clarifying process. My use of the English language became simpler, more accessible, and I learnt to make every word count.

At one point while I was in India, my mother became ill and I sent her a *yoga nidra* [deep relaxation] tape. Years later when I returned to Australia, she said to me, 'You know that tape you sent me from India? It's wearing out and I'd really like another one. Could you organise that?' She hadn't recognised that it was me who made the tape for her, and was talking on it! Recently, I was making another copy and I found the original tape. When I turned it on to listen, I stopped to question if it was actually me. I had developed such a distinctive South Indian accent!

If the language barrier was challenging, then it was countered by the openness and appreciation of the students. There was a lot of love and affection among the women, and I learnt an enormous amount from them. I was teaching them traditional yoga techniques and they were teaching me about Indian culture and mythology, the essential background of yoga. Where Swamiji's ashram brought about an immersion in yoga, my teaching led to an immersion in Indian culture. My students introduced me to stories from the old texts, to the traditional ways of preparing food and dressing, and to rituals such as temple and marriage ceremonies.

One of the benefits of studying in India was that the differences in culture continually challenged our assumptions—even with regards to everyday matters. For example, in Swamiji's ashram the cooking was done on a mud brick stove, which was a revelation to me because in Australia we cook on a gas or electric stove. But more than that, the kitchen was outside and the ground on which the food was prepared was mud washed with cow dung! I remember being called to the kitchen to help prepare a meal and seeing men and women sitting in a circle on the ground with a burlap sack in the middle, peeling the vegetables. Because of the cow-dung and mud floor, I went into this area wearing my thongs. The Indians were horrified! Shoes are worn outside on the road where there are parasites and dirt, but you do not bring your shoes into a house, certainly not into the kitchen-area. On the other hand, I was horrified that they were sitting around peeling vegetables on a mud and cowdung floor! Later someone explained to me that it is antiseptic and keeps the flies away. That sort of cultural contrast was constant.

My assumptions about how life should work were continually challenged, and this gave me a strong sense of cultural relativity. I questioned what it was that I had identified with. What supported my personal identity? This gave me a fresh perspective on what it might mean to be an Australian, and it helped me to break any unthinking identification with an Australian culture. (These identifications weren't necessarily negative—I recognised some very positive aspects to the Australian culture too.)

In Bangalore people frequently commented that in our ashram everyone was treated equally, regardless of class or caste. This is not true in India generally, where there are still a lot of caste divisions, but in the ashram people who would normally never sit next to each other would be seated side-by-side. And while this was a high yogic ideal, it was much easier for an Australian to implement, because we are brought up in a relatively egalitarian society. We were able to break down Indian caste distinctions without the emotional resistance that might have been there for Indian swamis.

Although born Australian, I never felt like an impostor in India studying a foreign tradition. Swami Satyananda would always emphasise that yoga is universal and is not restricted by religion or by culture. It is also part of yoga that the teachings are presented in a way appropriate to the times and to the cultural context. So yoga in the west has a slightly different flavour to yoga in the east. Even ashrams that follow the same tradition have slightly different flavours.

My experience in the ashram would be very hard to replicate today. I mean this literally, because not only is the old Bihar School of Yoga no longer used as the main ashram, but Swami Satyananda no longer takes *sannyas* training. Although *sannyas* training continues under Swami Niranjan, the Bihar School of Yoga has been transformed into Bihar Yoga Bharati, India's first yoga university. In Australia, there are Satyananda ashrams at Mangrove Mountain near Sydney, and Rocklyn near Melbourne, where students can sample a traditional ashram lifestyle. These ashrams did not exist when I left for India.

Back in 1974, Australians didn't need visas for India and you could stay as long as you liked. Over the years, trouble developed, in particular with the Sikh separatist movement which had a government-in-exile in London. A new policy was then introduced requiring Commonwealth passport holders to have a visa. When Mrs Gandhi was assassinated in 1985, the Indian government decided that all Commonwealth passport holders would have to leave the country because overseas Indian communities were implicated in supporting the separatist movement. I don't know how true any of that was, but the consequence was that we had to apply for visas. Our visas weren't extended and we were given what was called a Quit India notice. We had to leave.

As it happened, my Quit India notice came at exactly the time I was contemplating a change. I had been in India for nearly twelve years and I felt that I needed to move on somehow, but I didn't know how. During the seven years in Bangalore, I had been travelling around regularly. There was a town called Coimbatore where I would go three or four times a year to teach, and in the last year that I was in India, I left Bangalore and moved to Coimbatore to establish a yoga centre there.

One of the great things about living in India as part of a community was that I found many doors opened to me that were not normally open to westerners, certainly not to tourists. For example, I did a pilgrimage into the Himalayas with Indian people. So, when it came time to decide on my next step, I considered returning to the mountains north of India and losing myself there. But really, I wasn't sure what to do. I had my list of possible changes, and returning to Australia was right at the bottom. Then the cosmos stepped in. I had a series of very striking, very vivid dreams about leaving India. Next thing I knew, I received a telegram from the Indian government saying that they wouldn't renew my visa and that I had to leave the country and return to Australia.

# THIS IS YOGA?

After nearly twelve years in India, it was a test for me to come back to Australia. Not only was I changing cultures once again, I was leaving ashram life, leaving my work, my colleagues and dear friends—all at once. I went through a period of adjustment that allowed me to reflect on the efficacy of my training. Had it made me flexible in mind as well as in body? How readily did I adjust to being back in Australia, to finding a new direction in my life?

When I first went to India I almost expected to see people standing on their heads at the airport in Calcutta. What I found was that a lot of Indians do not practise yoga, despite being aware of it. Back in Australia, I knew that the Satyananda Yoga movement had grown quite strong in my absence, and that yoga generally had become more accepted in the west. But I also thought that people understood yoga in the way that I understood it. I was shocked to find that this was not so.

When I would say that I took yoga classes, people would ask, 'and do you teach meditation?' Yes! Of course! Meditation *is* yoga. Meditation is the essence of yoga, from my point of view, and from the point of view from which I was trained. It was a real surprise to come back and discover that most yoga classes were mainly about posture [*asana*], that most teachers said nothing about yoga philosophy, and that finding somewhere to learn meditation was extremely difficult. This led me to start up yoga classes in the Satyananda tradition, which included the full range of teachings: the postures, some yoga philosophy, some breathing [*pranayama*] and meditation training.

Just as teaching yoga in Bangalore had been about finding the most effective mode of communication, teaching in Australia was about demystifying my experiences and the yoga practices in order to connect with people. Yoga is about oneness, after all. I stopped wearing robes, for instance, because I felt that they created a separation between myself and the students, where what I was trying to convey was that yoga was about union. I wanted to make it clear that yoga is accessible to anyone but instead, people were focusing on the unusual experience I had had in India. I also gradually trained myself to stop using the Sanskrit names and use the English names of the practices. I didn't want separation; I wanted connection.

There are many varied reasons for being interested in yoga, all of them valid. When I came back to Australia I met a woman in her late seventies who had been a yoga teacher for forty years. She was someone I really respected, and her students were very serious yogis. She was critical of the fact that I was teaching yoga for therapeutic ends; she thought that was a debasement of yoga. I explained that people come to yoga because they have high blood pressure, or they have diabetes or they need stress management, but they often discover something else and you can't dismiss physical, therapeutic needs as a valid starting point. You can't know where people are going to go when they start and you can't pre-judge these things. When I first found yoga, something within me recognised it and I continued on with it—I don't think this trajectory is unique to me.

When I was in Bangalore I met a retired squadron leader. Air force pilots retire when they are about forty years old, as the defence force wants only really young, fit people—and so this man undertook yoga training to improve his heart fitness. He became so involved with yoga that he trained as a teacher with me in Bangalore, and then later took *sannyas* with Swami

Satyananda. His name now is Swami Anandmungle. When I had to leave India at the end of 1985, he was one of the people who helped continue the ashram in Bangalore. He has developed and expanded it and kept it running over all these years.

When I first returned to Australia, I did not want to continue day-to-day teaching of postures, breathing and meditation. Instead I was looking for a different way to be involved in yoga, so I went back to university and upgraded my qualifications to a Masters in psychology. When I did resume teaching, my main concern was to use my psychology training to support people's yoga practice.

When people come to yoga for stress management, they begin to relax very deeply, but they also begin to access the source of their stress, and they need support. If they feel too challenged by emotions that arise, they might retreat from the practice. I felt that psychological counselling was a way I could support people. For me, it was very much secondary to yoga teaching, but it was a way to work through the emotional material that was coming up for people in their yoga practice.

In India, the structure of the society and the culture prepare you for the emotional difficulty that usually accompanies commitment to an inner practice. Such traditional societies *are* more conservative, but they also provide traditional and ritualised ways of working through difficult feelings, like loss or grief. When you are practising yoga in a culture outside of India where tradition and ritual have fallen away, where the religious structure has faded, and where family structures are rapidly changing, and have been changing for several generations, you don't have the kind of practical or philosophical support for the emotional problems you may encounter in your practice, or in life in general.

# STILLNESS OF MIND, STEADINESS OF SPIRIT

At the invitation of other teachers and organisations, I began sharing some of the more esoteric teachings of yoga. People from different parts of Australia asked me to come and teach— these were mainly existing yoga teachers who wanted to explore more fully the intricacies of teaching meditation to students. Swami Niranjan was encouraging of that and I saw it as part of my contribution to Swamiji's mission of taking 'yoga from door to door and shore to shore'.

One of the things I discovered was that a lot of yoga teachers who hadn't had much access to the traditional teachings felt fearful of teaching meditation because they hadn't experienced it themselves. They didn't fully know what it involved and were a little afraid of what such a practice might awaken in themselves and their students. And this is true: you cannot teach meditation effectively if you don't have experience of it. This is true for yoga teaching in general, but particularly true of these more subtle areas. You have to explore the territory yourself first.

I also became aware that there were students whose yoga practice had brought them to the point of wanting to explore meditation, and that they had started to do Buddhist meditation because they didn't know that yoga had its own rich tradition of meditation practice.

In Australia in the late eighties and early nineties there were plenty of weekend yoga retreats on offer, but they were not structured around meditation. A typical retreat would include classes on postures and breathing, together with karma yoga [selfless service]. Sometimes there would be *kirtan* [group singing of Sanskrit mantras and hymns] in the evenings.

Meditation was restricted to short relaxation practices such as *yoga nidra*, and silence was not observed except occasionally for short periods, before breakfast, for example.

The most popular form of Buddhist meditation retreat was Goenka-style Vipassana, one of which I attended in 1986, and it could not have offered a greater contrast to Satyananda-style yoga. Goenka retreats are ten days long and meditation is practised for up to ten hours a day, interrupted only by breaks for meals and brief walks. Silence is observed for the whole ten days, men and women are segregated at all times, and communication by any means, including eye contact, is banned. A videotaped instruction on how to witness sensation in the body by S.N. Goenka is shown every evening [S.N. Goenka founded Vipassana retreats in India in 1969]. The practice of *asana* is explicitly banned, along with tai chi, reading, writing, the repetition of mantras and the use of *malas* [prayer beads]. The rules are very strict, but a great many people report benefits from the experience.

How had this apparent gulf between yoga and Buddhist meditation come to pass?

The most common manifestation of yoga in the west has been Hatha yoga joined with a brief relaxation practice, devoid of meditation. The schools of Buddhism that came to the west came with a strong tradition of meditation teaching, but generally viewed yoga as a lesser path. Buddhists who wanted to incorporate yoga into their practice would typically be accused of 'spiritual shopping'.

It appears that this split between Buddhism and yoga—which still persists among many practitioners—stems from a long Buddhist tradition. It is said to date back to the Buddha himself, who taught that the yoga practices he had followed—

*asana, pranayama,* advanced yoga meditation techniques, and especially extreme aesthetic practices—did not by themselves lead to enlightenment. This teaching was misinterpreted over the centuries to mean that only meditation was required for enlightenment. In the twentieth century, yoga was interpreted in the west as *asana* and *pranayama,* Buddhism as meditation.

For Buddhist practitioners, this meant that their meditation was denied all the wonderful benefits of the yogic preparation for meditation. As a result, many Buddhist meditators told me they suffered considerable physical pain during their 'sits'. Although there is one school of Buddhism that uses pain as the main focus of meditation, pain prevents most meditators from accessing the deeper levels of meditation. In extreme cases, long hours of sitting in meditation caused people to injure their spine and joints.

For western yoga practitioners, this historical split meant that they were deprived of the meditation experiences their practices had primed them for. In India, however, the yoga tradition has always included a strong emphasis on meditation. Patanjali's famous yoga text, the *Yoga Sutras,* is adamant that the purpose of *asana* and *pranayama* is preparation for meditation.

One of Swami Satyananda's great achievements was to restore meditation to western yoga. His 1974 book, *Meditations from the Tantras,* is a testament to this.

In 1994, eight years after I returned to Australia, I began teaching traditional yoga meditation retreats. (I have since handed them over to other teachers.) These were intensive one-week residential retreats where students could explore ways of building a yoga practice that was tailored to powerfully move them into meditation. These traditional meditation retreats were based on the yogic model: *pranayama, mudra* and *bandha* would lead into several sittings of meditation each day, which were in turn supported by *asana*. Silence was kept the whole time. I included *dharma* [code of spiritual living] talks, and a written question and answer time. There was plenty of opportunity for participants to explore the various practices and to find the sequence of practices that was most effective in leading them into meditation. As well as this, there was the support to *be with* what arose in meditation.

Nobody has a perfectly aligned spine or perfect posture, and aches and pains are inevitable during long meditation sessions, even when sessions are broken by yoga postures. In response to this I developed a kind of yoga therapy: a fifteen to twenty-minute sequence of yoga practices that I called 'Meditator's First Aid'. I subsequently taught this at all my yoga retreats and also at a couple of Buddhist retreats that I co-taught with a Vipassana teacher. Many students found it effective and it is still taught at yoga and Buddhist meditation retreats around Australia.

## MEDITATION AND KARMA YOGA

There are many ways to meditate, and Satyananda yoga emphasises finding the right technique for each person, rather than one practice for all. Whatever the technique, meditation helps develop concentration and focus, clarity and insight. It allows for exploration of those more subtle dimensions of our being of which we may not be aware but that still impinge on our day-to-day life. The awareness that we cultivate 'on the cushion' we then carry with us into the rest of our lives.

This is the essence of Karma yoga: extending our meditative

practice into the rest of life so that all of our life becomes a kind of meditation. Issues come up in our relationships with other people or in our work that don't come up on the meditation cushion. They show us aspects of ourselves that would be overlooked if all we did was meditate. When they do come up, we can then take them back to our cushion. This interrelationship between our meditation practice and our life is a constant. In this way, life becomes more interesting and also more insightful.

In our formal sitting meditation we deepen the subtle awareness of who we really are and then attempt to remain aware of that in all aspects of life. By bringing depth of awareness into every moment, we become more fully alive and each moment becomes richer, tastier. Whatever we are doing can become part of our path of self-understanding and self-growth.

When I first worked in the ashram press, I was very bored. Learning to come to terms with boredom is about learning to be fully alive in the moment and not to overlay it with expectations. When you start to do that, you taste the flavour of each moment and you do not get bored, not even if the activity is unappealing to you.

Yoga means 'yoking'—joining what has separated, making one whole. It involves integration and implies integrity. Integrity means bringing to any situation not just my physical self and not just my mind, but the whole of myself. At times we may be aware of our bodies but not the workings of our minds, at other times we may be aware of mind and thought—and yet meditation shows us that there is something beyond these two states as well. There are further dimensions to the human being, and the traditional aim of yoga is to expand our awareness in order to explore those. All the challenges we face in our practice and in life allow us to discover the full potential of humanity, and to discover our own essence. As we become more aware of our own unique essence, we also become aware of our profound connection with others and the universe. And this, yogis tell us in the old texts, brings such light into our lives that 'it makes everything shine'.

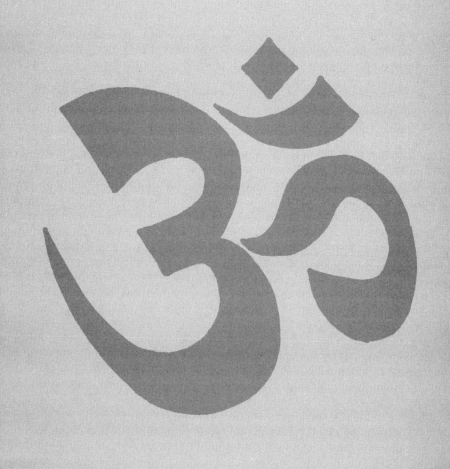

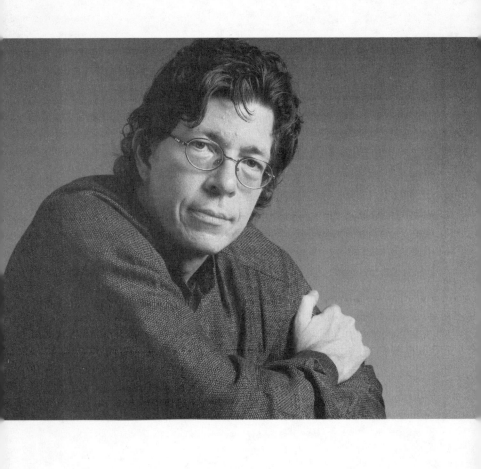

# 5

# KNOW YOURSELF, KNOW THE SELF

*Robert  E.  Svoboda*

*What is the purpose of being born? To recognise yourself, to realise that you are neither the body nor the mind but rather the Eternal Soul which is the Ultimate Unity.*

Vimalananda

Robert E. Svoboda

*At eighteen years old, the same young age that most people graduate from high school, Robert Svoboda was accepting his undergraduate degree in science and enrolling for the next, medicine, when he decided to pause and see a little of the world. He left America on a one-year ticket intending to visit exotic destinations, but what he ultimately saw was life itself afresh—the journey became never-ending.*

*When the twelve months were up his plans to return home were abandoned, but not his desire to study. Instead of becoming a doctor in the United States he moved to Bombay and in 1980 graduated from the Tilak Ayurveda Mahavidyalaya, University of Pune, becoming the first westerner to gain qualifications in Ayurveda [traditional Indian medicine] from an Indian university. He won all but one of the year's awards.*

*It was the 'other' education he received in India, earned outside the realm of institutions, for which he has attracted out-of-the-ordinary attention. While a student in Bombay, Robert met his mentor, Vimalananda, who introduced him to yoga, Jyotisha [Vedic astrology] and Tantra [a form of yoga], as well as ushering him into the world of Aghora [an extreme and little-known form of Tantra]. An Aghori [one who practises Aghora] meditates in cemeteries in the middle of the night, and engages in other seemingly strange practices in order to penetrate the illusory appearance of life and perceive its universal essence. Robert explains this pathway in compelling detail in his most famous book, Aghora: At the Left Hand of God, which is the first in a trilogy that chronicles his unusual time with Vimalananda and some of the teachings. The central philosophy of Aghora, as with most schools of yoga, is oneness—the nature of all existence is universal—which gives rise to Vimalananda's pithy summation of the purpose of spiritual practice: 'Everywhere I see, everything is Me.'*

*On the afternoon that we meet to discuss yoga there is no evidence of a loincloth, no trident, not even a skull and crossbones to be seen.*

*As if in contrast to the image of the terrifying cemetery-dwelling Aghori, Robert's skin is milky like a newborn's and his eyes are pools of blue-green that seem awake with wonder. If his manner is unexpectedly gentle and approachable then, predictably, his intellect towers.*

*Robert is the author of twelve books and numerous articles on Ayurveda, yoga and related topics. Since leaving India in 1986 he has travelled the world constantly to consult, teach, study and lecture. During the conversation he sips steaming rooibos tea from South Africa, his long fingers gripped, tentacle-like, by rings of metal, shell and precious stone. He explains how yoga offers a means to fully understand one's true nature and, in so doing, to live each moment of life 'better'.*

## THE ROAD TO BOMBAY

Am I an Aghori? I would not use that word for myself. A real Aghori is someone who effortlessly makes no distinction between Ganges water and gutter water, as they would say in India, or between *tiramisu* and trash, and I am not quite at that stage.

Am I a yogi? Again, I wouldn't apply that word to myself. Of course, yoga can be defined in different ways. Patanjali, the author of the *Yoga Sutras*, defined yoga as *citta vrtti nirodhah*—which means, a restraint of the fluctuations of the mind. But I prefer Krishna's definition in the *Bhagavad Gita*. Krishna's definition, which is found in Chapter II, verse 50, is '*Yogah karmasu kaushalam*'. 'Yoga is adeptness in action.' Let me explain.

There is a particular kind of sacred grass in India called *kusha* grass that people use to make mats to sit on in meditation and in rituals. When it is dry this *kusha* grass is very sharp and you can easily slice yourself with it. Those who are said to be *kaushala* can handle that grass without slicing their hands. Therefore the word *kaushalam* can mean 'expertise'. It can also mean 'ease'. If you can handle life in a similar way, handle even those parts of life that are sharp without gouging yourself, then to me that is what yoga is all about. As Hemingway said, 'grace under pressure'. Yoga is very much about living with grace under pressure.

My mentor would say, 'Yoga is meant to make every home a happy home.' So would I think of myself as a yogi? I would think of myself as someone who is practising yoga and attempting to get to the stage of being in a position to always handle every situation gracefully.

Circumstances led me to view life this way. When I was young I was in a hurry to finish formal schooling. I was able to graduate with a bachelor's degree from the University of Oklahoma when I was eighteen. Then I didn't know what to do, so I thought that I might as well go to medical school. The only school that would admit me, because I was young, was in Oklahoma where I was living at the time. I got admitted there and I thought that I would first take a trip to a distant place that was very exotic before I had to go back and stay in the lab for six or seven years. I went to Africa.

I crossed Africa overland from the west coast to the east coast and when I got to Kenya I participated in an ethnographic expedition with the National Museum of Kenya. Circumstances were such that I ended up being ritually initiated into the tribe that we were studying, becoming the first white member of the Pokot tribe of northern Kenya. I was very proud of this until recently when I was visiting a friend who lives in Jaipur in India, who had a couple friends staying from Kenya. When I told them I was a Pokot they started to laugh. I had to ask why exactly they were laughing and I was told that the Pokot are best known in Kenya for being cattle rustlers. I thought, 'Great, so this is what I have been so proud of for the last thirty years! I went from being Texan, the home of cattle rustlers in America, to the Pokot, renowned for cattle rustling in Africa!'

Once I was in Africa I decided that I was not quite ready to go home, so I managed to postpone going to medical college for one year, then flew to England, travelled overland to Nepal, went on a couple of treks, and then made my way down the Himalayas to Bodhgaya, in Eastern India. There, in January 1974, the Dalai Lama was giving a *Kalachakra* [Tantric practices to raise awareness] initiation, which I attended. Afterwards I thought, 'This yoga business is really very good. I must study it.'

I ended up in Bombay and I was literally at the right place at just the right time. I met someone who introduced me to somebody, who introduced me to somebody, who introduced me to somebody who got me into the Ayurvedic College [Tilak Ayurveda Mahavidyalaya] in Pune, where I then lived and studied from 1974 to 1980.

I met Vimalananda, my mentor, in 1975. After college I lived in Bombay from 1982 to 1986, living with Vimalananda for the first two years. He left his body in December of 1983. I continued on there for a couple of years and then I started spending more time in the United States. And now I have no fixed address. Since 1986, I have spent three or four months of every year in India, a couple of months in North America, a month in Europe, as well as visiting other places. Lately I have been cutting down my time in India to spend more time in Texas with my mother who is eighty-seven years old and until recently was still teaching Sunday School.

My parents' faith influenced me strongly as I grew up, and

I still regularly worship Jesus Christ as my *kula devata*, my family deity. Only now the practices I mainly follow are derived from the Tantric tradition, and a little of the *Aghora* tradition. Yes, when I go to Benares, I do regularly sit in the cemetery, and make fire offerings. I have performed rituals with human bones and skulls and such things. These are all *Aghora* practices. I never had the desire to get involved with this set of bizarre practices, but my mentor knew this was the direction I needed to go in, and set me on this path. I am by no means as adept as my mentor, who could do all manner of very weird and wonderful practices, but I try to do what I have the aptitude for.

That is what I think yoga is all about: doing what you are able to do in the best possible way, rather than having some kind of pre-concocted image of how things *should* be, and then trying to manoeuvre yourself into the procrustean bed of your own image. I think that's where a lot of people stray.

What a good mentor should be able to do—because there are plenty of bad mentors too—is look at you and decide what sort of life should be best for you. Suppose the mentor looks at you and sees that, in fact, even if you would like to get married, there is no way in hell that you will be able to make your marriage work, then you are better off doing something different. If, on the other hand, the mentor sees that you are better off living in the middle of the city and sharing your knowledge and your expertise with a group of people that you are going to find there, then he or she is better off explaining that to you in clear and unambiguous terms.

The basic reason for having a mentor is to have someone whose energy will continue to travel with you during this life and on into the next. A mentor's energy will travel with you, will provide you with something outside of yourself that you can rely on. That gives you something to have faith in. Having faith in something means having a point from which you can proceed outwards and to which you can return. It is always good to have a centre. This is what the mentor should do: provide you with a centre. Whether that is the mentor himself or whether that is a big rock that you focus on, or Lord Shiva, or a rockmelon doesn't matter. What matters is that it acts as something that you can use as your centre, and then that centre is something towards which you can aspire.

## ASPIRING TO WHOLENESS

Ask yourself: What do I have faith in? How do I make this manifest in my life? To make what you have faith in manifest regularly is to build a spiritual practice. I think that the most meaningful practices are ones that have not been prescribed, but are things that you develop on your own.

Should you have a trusted friend who always gives you good advice, you would be wise to meet that friend on a regular basis. Similarly, it is a good habit to sit regularly with whomever you regard as your mentor, or centre. If you have an affinity for one of the *devas* [divine entities] like Shiva or Ganesha, or for an incarnation of the divine like Jesus Christ, or for a representative of the divine who is now living like His Holiness the Dalai Lama, it would be easy to use that as a point on which you focus.

Take His Holiness the Dalai Lama, for example, as many people have an affinity for him. Even though when you sit with him it appears that you are focusing on him, really you are focusing *through* him. He is the lens through which you are bringing reality into sharper focus. His Holiness has been kind enough to consent to serve, on the one hand, as a focus for people who are aspiring to Spirit [all-pervading, omnipresent essence] and, on the other hand, also as a vehicle for the descent of Spirit into manifestation. In particular, the aspect of Spirit that he has specialised in is compassion, because he acts as a vehicle for the force that the Buddhists call *Avalokiteshvara*. *Avalokshena* means 'to look down'. *Avalokiteshvara* means the Buddha that looks down upon humanity with compassion. One of the reasons *Avalokiteshvara* is able to do that is because people like His Holiness the Dalai Lama are available to act as his representative, a person through whom the energy of compassion can project itself.

So if you meet with His Holiness on a regular basis—on a daily basis in meditation, let's say—you will develop and cultivate your relationship with that aspect of reality and that aspect of reality can then educate you about other aspects of reality. His Holiness becomes the representative of the totality of all realities, of The Reality, at the moment that you worship him. In the same way that you are not the finite characteristics that you represent, that you have self-identified with, he is not the finite set of characteristics that he represents. He acts at that moment as the interface between limited and unlimited, and you are helping to make him into that interface. In this way he will appreciate what you are doing for him because your identifying with him in this way actually facilitates his experiencing of this reality. His Holiness acts as a gateway, by virtue of having the energy of various people focusing on him, *through* him, to *Avalokiteshvara*, and by virtue of having the energy of *Avalokiteshvara* come through him towards these people. In a sense, he is acting as the Internet Service Provider, because the

Net is out there and you are over here but you have to connect somehow.

This is one way to aspire towards Spirit. As my mentor used to say, when you talk about identifying with Spirit, you are talking about identifying with the absolute totality of all existence. He would say, 'Personally, it is very difficult for me to self-identify with the sun, much less our solar system or the galaxy, which is one galaxy out of billions of galaxies.' This is why he always recommended the multi-step method. Do the little things first. Know yourself in order to know the Self.

## KNOWING THE SELF IS TO KNOW THE SELF

There are philosophical systems that say that the material world is totally corrupt and evil, that Spirit is perfect and pure, and that the two are totally separate from one another [known as dualism]. Then there are other philosophical systems, including the one I espouse, which says that if something is generated out of something that is perfect, then it also has to be perfect. This is what people refer to when they talk about Advaita Vedanta [non-dualist Vedic philosophy].

Most people who talk about Advaita Vedanta are talking about Shankaracharya's approach [an eighth-century celebrated sage], which says that only the Ultimate Reality is real, and that the reality of this world is 'erroneous', unreal. The variety of Advaita Vedanta that I like far better, is the version that comes to us from Vallabhacharya [a sixteenth-century sage], who talks about 'One in all, and all in One' [that is, the microcosm reflected in the macrocosm and the macrocosm reflected in the microcosm].

119

He says that the 'one' (Absolute Consciousness) is always present in the 'all' (that is, the multiplicity of our world). The all is also always present in the One. The Self, capital S, is omnipresent, and the many individual copies of the self, lower case 's', are also real and existent—the relationship between the two is also real.

The idea, then, that spirituality somehow involves you getting from a point in the world of name and form, to a point of reunion with the Absolute, is only one way of expressing the potential result of a spiritual path. Some may not desire to end up *there*, instead of *here*. None of the world's great devotees ever wanted to end up *becoming* what they were focusing on.

Take Krishna and Radha [Krishna's divine consort]. Radha wouldn't enjoy herself if she were to get completely dissolved into Krishna; there would be no excitement left, no lovemaking anymore. She'd be gone; they'd be reunited. So these two entities maintain a degree of separation, uniting only to separate again, and separating only again to be reunited. Union. Separation. Union. Separation. Many people say this is not spiritual, that the only definition of spirituality and mysticism is to proceed to the Reality of non-dualism, to redissolve into the Absolute. But why should there be no other definition of spirituality than this? I don't see Nature as so linear and uni-dimensional that simple redissolution should be the only Reality, and neither does Indian tradition.

After all, from the point of view of Ayurveda and *Jyotisha*, the human being is a *pinda* [embryo], a microcosm of the big macrocosm. Everything that is happening out there is happening in here. If there is the possibility out in the universe for the Self to experience itself, then there is the possibility in the internal universe also. In fact, that is why they say the body and the universe were created in the first place, so they could act as a mirror through which the Ultimate Reality could visualise itself.

We can think of the Ultimate Self as being 'up there' in the sense of it being so rarefied that it has no limitations whatsoever. As it projects itself 'down' into manifestation it takes on characteristics that limit it progressively, level by level, until you get to where we currently are, sitting at the bottom of a pile of limitations. If you had the desire, and the right alignment, you could proceed directly back towards the Self—and we would all wave goodbye to you, and wish you *bon voyage!*

## FIRST THINGS FIRST

Modern life encourages people to leak their energy into the environment all the time. Advertising is trying to grab your attention, so it can collect your money, and personal information, and suchlike. Most people are very much a part of this system, which is kind of like *The Matrix*: a system that is sucking the life and juice out of people, throwing them a bone to gnaw on now and again. Most people stay in this condition because they have been lured—they are thinking in the direction of the system, salivating in its direction while being dragged towards it. There is no centre anymore. People have nothing to relate to anymore.

To align oneself, we start with the simplest things first. I like to point out that as the years go by you are not really getting older you are getting less young, which means that your body doesn't respond as well as it used to. When things go wrong they take longer to come back into balance. Even when you are young and it appears that you have unlimited energy, it is just *maya* [the illusion of existence]. You will in fact run out of energy at some point. It is good to learn while you are young to use your energy in energy-efficient ways.

One efficient way to use your energy, for instance, is to learn that if you cannot digest milk then you are better off not drinking it. Even though it says in the scriptures that milk is very *sattvic* [harmonising] and that if you eat *sattvic* food your mind will become more subtle, and the more subtle your mind becomes the closer you will get to the spiritual life. But if you don't digest milk properly you are creating big problems for yourself that will negate whatever quantum of *sattva* you might get out of the milk by the more practical real world experience of indigestion. This is why Ayurveda in particular says: Do all of the simple things first. Don't do the simple things later. Do them first. Get up at the right time every day. Get enough sleep. Get enough exercise. Make sure that the digestive tract is working. Make sure that you breathe properly.

A lot of people say, 'Oh yeah! I definitely want to be a spiritual person,' and they have a small, restricted idea of what a spiritual person should look like. A spiritual person has a pentagram over the door. A spiritual person buys sandalwood incense. And spiritual people very much like to consume the fragrance of beautiful flowers, like lilies: so this is the good part of being a spiritual person. The not-so-good part is that yes, sometimes your partner does not act spiritually enough. And everyone else fails to act spiritually from time to time too—how inconvenient is that? You, on the other hand, are perfectly spiritual.

Yoga is very much about you identifying who you are. What things has your ego identified with? Some things are obvious to you—like your name—and some things are less obvious to you—decisions you may have made when you were very small that you are no longer conscious of, or ways in which you are deceiving yourself in order to permit yourself to act in other ways. The clearer you can identify who you are, the easier it is going to be for you to establish a vision of what you can do with yourself, and then to actualise that vision.

Here is where things like astrology are handy. You want to look in the horoscope and see very practical things. An old friend of mine who is a professor of Sanskrit was asking about his wife who is also an academic but who wanted to get into the healing profession. I know her and it didn't seem like she would be very fit for that kind of thing, then I looked at her horoscope and that didn't encourage things either, then I asked a mutual friend of ours who also has a good perspective on astrology and she didn't see anything either. While it was certainly possible that she might enter into the healing profession, it didn't look very likely. It looked like the amount of energy she would need for that kind of transformation would not be commensurate with the result.

You can also use Ayurveda as a tool of self-knowledge. How does my organism work? What is my physical constitution? What are the limits that my constitution imposes on me? If you are an extremely over-*pitta*-ised person [*pitta* is an Ayurvedic constitution dominated by fire and water] are you going to be happy living in extremely hot, humid weather? No, you will not; that question need not be asked, because that sort of life will definitely not work for you. These are all practical ways of knowing your small, personal self, so that you can know the Self, that Self that is both different from you, but also the same.

# A WORD ABOUT ASANA

Yoga is a practical experiment that you can do with yourself, but you must accomplish it within the context of the rest of your life—how can you separate your yoga from the rest of your life, when the very word 'yoga' means 'to yoke together, to unite'? Sanskrit texts always assume that you will remember what was mentioned beforehand. Yoga texts discuss the *yamas* and *niyamas* [moral observances and self restraints] before they talk about *asana* and *pranayama*, which in turn are discussed before *pratyahara, dharana, dhyana,* and *samadhi* [sensory withdrawals, one-pointed focus, concentration, ecstatic absorption]. This means that at each later stage—*asana, pranayama, pratyahara* and so on—you need to follow the principles of the earlier stages, beginning with the *yamas* and *niyamas: svadhyaya* [self-study], *ishvara pranidhana* [surrender to Spirit], *shaucha* [purity], and so on.

*Asana* can certainly be a valuable part of yoga, provided that you don't try to limit yoga to being *asana*. A surprising number of people—surprising, at least, to me—get into yoga, and think of yoga solely as *asana*. They don't think much about how yoga is very concerned with practical things, like your way of interacting with the world. This misconception that 'yoga is *asana*' happens because the average yoga teacher doesn't mention the *yamas* and the *niyamas*—and those who do, usually do so only in passing, before proceeding directly to *asana*. What they don't realise—because they haven't been properly taught themselves—is that the *yamas* and *niyamas* are the attitudes that also apply to your *asana* practice.

So the *yamas—ahimsa* [non-violence], *satya* [truth], *asteya* [non-stealing], *bramacharya* [integrity in thought and action], *aparigraha* [non-covetousness]—apply to your *asana* practice. For example, just because you can see that someone else can do another *asana* better than you, do not covet what they are able to do. Rather, if you acknowledge that you are different from them and they are different from you, you observe *ahimsa* [non-violence]. You don't perform violence on yourself and damage yourself because you are trying to reach some end point that you have identified as *the* end point, but which may have nothing to do with the real end point. *Ahimsa* is not just about behaving in thought and action without violence in regards to anyone else, it starts with yourself.

*Asana* comes from a Sanskrit word that means 'to sit'. My mentor used to say that in his day the way people were trained to sit was to go inside a room and close the door, and there they would be. Once a day people would bring you food, but there were no phones, no books, nothing to distract you, just you and the room. At the end of six months you would know how to sit. Baba Hari Dass, who is a yogi who lives in the United States now, says that when he was studying yoga, a guru would make you sit in a comfortable *asana* and fill your lap with dirt and sow seeds and come back to see if, when the seeds had sprouted, they were pointed straight up. If they were, you knew how to sit. Most people today have great trouble sitting. Why try doing all kinds of fancy, dynamic *asana* before you can sit?

Another meaning of *asana* is that not only should you be able to sit, but the *prana* [life's energy] in your body should be able to sit too. You should be able to get the *prana* in your body to be well seated in your body. If your vigorous physical activity causes you to pant, then your *prana* is not well seated. The more that you get out of breath, the more you are transforming *prana* into *vata*. The difference between *prana* and *vata* is that *prana* is well centred in the body and therefore it can be calm. *Vata* has lost its connection to the centre, and thus its ability to calm down. It becomes nervous energy, which can only be burned off. *Asana* practice that is overactive will most likely set you up for some sort of trouble. One of the problems with *asana* practice, as it exists—let's not call it 'yoga' when it is nothing more than *asana* practice—is that it can overstimulate the *prana* in your system. *Prana* that is aligned moves easily and freely and is not overly stimulated.

When people go into studying yoga-as-*asana* practice, outside any other context, it is quite natural that they will start to think of it in terms of stretch and strength development and muscular development. What they are doing when they do that is directing the *prana* in the body to activate the physical body, to activate the part of the organism that is pretty much the lower, if not the lowest, part. So if Spirit is something that is rarefied and refined, and if, instead, you put your energy into something that is very dense and heavy, then that will create problems for you. You may not notice it initially, but eventually a certain level of cognitive dissonance develops within your ego.

Your ego is always trying to determine the path you should pursue. It does this in order to gain an idea of the pattern it can follow while disconnecting from certain parts of you and reconnecting to other parts—a process that is happening all the time. You started off as the child of your parents, and were mainly the child of your parents up until the age of eighteen or twenty. Thereafter, you might define yourself in relation to your spouse or partner. We humans are very social animals, we like to define and redefine ourselves *vis-à-vis* other humans. Redefinition is happening all the time, but the ego likes to have an idea of what the overall picture looks like. So if you are always saying to yourself, 'I am identifying with my body', eventually you are going to have a problem, if no sooner than at the time that you die, because your body, we can be sure, is not coming with you then. This doesn't mean that you have to disconnect from *everything* early on: that might not be 'adept action'.

To me, the aim of *sadhana* is to self-identify with Spirit, to move into a healthy relationship with Spirit. A spiritual practice should thus produce, if not a direct connection to Spirit, at least an aspiration to Spirit at all times. Therefore, it is worth considering, when you are doing your *asana* practice, are you extending yourself outwards and upwards towards Spirit? Or are you focusing mainly on what is going on with your little toe?

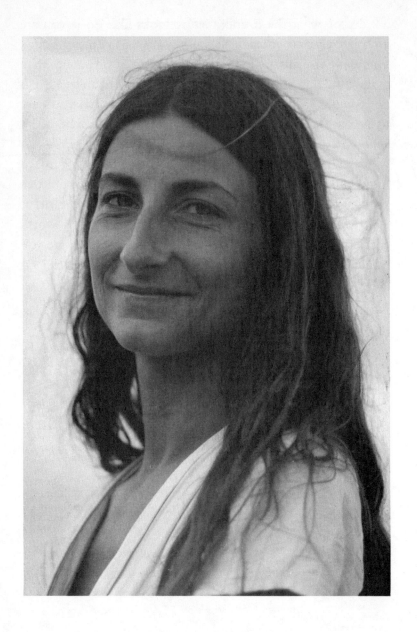

# 6

# FOLLOW YOUR DEEP, DRIVING DESIRE

## *Rose Baudin*

*I went to the woods because I wished to live deliberately, to front only the essential facts of life, and see if I could not learn what it had to teach, and not, when I came to die, discover that I had not lived.*

Henry David Thoreau

'Summa iru. *Tamil. Simply be.*' *He wagged his head village style from side to side in the way which meant a variety of things. 'If you can stop your mind and simply be you'll have no problems. Just sit quietly here, simply be . . . Do one thing at a time and do it properly. Sit properly, eat properly. Be properly. That means no wondering about what is going to happen at the temple, good or bad, or about what has happened. You're not there or there.' The cigar pointed behind to the tea stall and ahead to the estuary. 'Know where you are and be there.'*

*This passage from the novel* Earthman *written by Maggi Lidchi in the sixties would parallel a real life encounter between a young seeker Rose Baudin and her guru Swami Gauribala (the inspiration for the above character) that was soon to unfold.*

*In the early seventies, Rose-Ellen Rockermann, a young New Yorker barely out of school, quit her job on Madison Avenue, packed her bags and set off on a road trip with her boyfriend. Where they were headed was unclear, but why was certain. Rose-Ellen was on a quest to seek out 'men of wisdom' who would help her understand life and the truth behind existence.*

*Her quest led her to a farmhouse in Maine, through Asia, and eventually to the small island of Sri Lanka that hangs like a tailbone off the spine of India. There, she found her guru. Swami Gauribala of Jaffna was not a saintly Sri Lankan sadhu, as she had imagined she might find, but a mischievous twinkling-eyed German who wore only a sarong, snowy beard, smoky cigar and two strange words tattooed to the soft belly of his inner arm—*summa iru. *These words were the essence of his teaching and their meaning—'simply be'— would soon become clear. Swiftly, he disarmed his student of preconceptions she harboured about spirituality and armed her instead with essential teachings that would guide her on the journey within.*

*For the next sixteen years, Rose (as she became known) lived between the jungle of Sri Lanka and the beaches and mountains of India, alternating between studying with her guru and then attempting to make sense of the lessons within the context of her everyday life.*

*Like his student, Swami Gauribala, had too, left his home years earlier to embark on what he reportedly called his 'grail quest'. He left Germany in the thirties, going to Sri Lanka (then Ceylon) where he took robes in the Buddhist Island Hermitage. He was interned in India during World War II and afterwards led a nomadic life searching, similarly, for men of wisdom. He returned to Sri Lanka where he would finally meet his own guru, Yogaswami.*

*According to those who knew Swami Gauribala, his* sadhana *[spiritual practice] was extraordinary—he walked the two-month pilgrimage to the sacred jungle temple of Kataragama twenty-five times. In his lifetime he had acquired great depth of understanding and out-of-the-ordinary powers [siddhis], all of which he presented in the most down-to-earth of ways to those who knew him.*

*Rose now teaches yoga in the spirit and lineage of her guru. She is based in Australia and regularly conducts retreats in French Polynesia and America, as well as going on pilgrimage in India and making regular trips to Sri Lanka to continue her path and remain connected to the* parampara *[the lineage of spiritual energy and teachings passed from guru to disciple]. She talks about how her single-minded desire to seek the Truth, and to live among men who could help her find it, changed her life irrevocably and in ways she hadn't foreseen.*

*When I meet with her for our interview, Rose is sitting cross-legged on the timber deck that juts off her 'treehouse' home and overhangs a syrupy, lush tropical garden. Her eyes are a brilliant piercing green, her hair a long chestnut mane, and her skin golden like honey. She dares and charms with her exuberant energy as she recalls her story.*

# ꞏ꞉ LIVE AMONG MEN OF WISDOM

From a very young age, the burning desire that has driven me in this lifetime has been to discover what freedom really means and to live in a truly authentic way. I couldn't say that as a child I was walking around consciously looking for the guru, but in my heart I always longed to meet someone who could act as a guide and point me in the direction of truth and authenticity. This was my heart's deepest desire. As it says in the Upanishads [ancient yogic text]: 'You are what your deep, driving desire is. As your desire is, so is your will. As your will is, so is your deed. As your deed is, so is your destiny.' And so my life unfolded.

I grew up in an affluent, conservative community fifteen miles outside New York City, and yet, despite a privileged lifestyle, I observed that so many of us living there did not exude life's energy. Even as a young girl, I felt disturbed by the general atmosphere of society that seemed to lack joyful spontaneity. I questioned people's authenticity. I witnessed behaviour among people who held high positions in local politics and in the business world that did not inspire confidence in me. I felt disconcerted. The disillusionment increased after a four-year period working in New York City: first for a publishing company, then for a law firm on Fifth Avenue, and again for another publishing house on Madison Avenue. My experiences there caused me to lose respect for those in powerful positions whom most people admired, or feared. For the life of me, I could not understand their morality. I wanted to understand what *true* morality was and I sensed that this would not happen if I were to blindly follow the path that lay ahead of me. Instead, I set out hoping to find someone or something to point me in the direction of wisdom.

I quit my job and went off to explore the world. My boyfriend, Jon Hawley, and I criss-crossed North America several times before we settled down on a property in Maine, and it was there that I first began to submerge myself in yoga. Like so many at that time, I read *Autobiography of a Yogi*, which inspired me to become a member of the Self-Realization Fellowship and to study, via correspondence, Kriya yoga [taught by the Self-Realization Fellowship and emphasising meditation]. Already vegetarian, I went vegan, started practising *asana, pranayama* and meditation (as set out by SRF), observing one day of silence and one day of fasting every week.

The effects of the practices and austerities were so profound that they kindled in me a passion to plunge further into yoga philosophy. I studied the *Yoga Sutras* of Patanjali and although I soaked up its essence like a sponge, so much still eluded me! The resonance I felt with the *Sutras* stimulated my appetite for more, and so during our one year in Maine, with ten feet of snow and sub-zero temperatures during the winter months, there was nothing to do but practise, read sacred texts and feed both the inner and external fires.

This was the late sixties, early seventies and Baba Ram Dass [American yogi and author] had just come onto the scene with *Be Here Now*, his now-famous book on Indian spirituality. Ram Dass had met his guru in India, and so inspiring was his devotion that my boyfriend and I decided to sell up and follow that lead. So after spending a year submerging ourselves in yoga practices on our secluded property in Maine, we voyaged to India. Our journey led us to Sri Lanka and this is how I met my guru. Quite by chance.

One afternoon, my boyfriend and I were sitting on a beach in Colombo watching the sunset when seemingly out of nowhere a Sri Lankan man we had never met before, approached us. We didn't engage in much small talk. This man, whose name we learnt was Manik Sangrasagra, simply told us that there was going to be an extraordinary human being in Colombo that night and it would be our only chance to meet him. He gave us the address and left.

Although my deepest yearning was to meet a great man of knowledge, it is also in my nature to be somewhat timid and cautious. I didn't know what to do with this information. While my outward, surface tendency was to treat with caution the unknown, on a deeper level I will push through any fear or obstacle in order to remain tenaciously on the path to Truth. And so, despite my initial hesitation and misgivings, later that night we indeed went to the home of an Englishman named Mike Wilson (who later became Swami Siva Kalki) and it was there that I met the German, Swami Gauribala.

Mike Wilson's house appeared mysterious and archaic to me (especially coming from New Jersey!). It was enormous and impressive. It was brimming with all kinds of exotic artefacts and paraphernalia that made it look more like some arcane museum than a home. Covering one wall was an ancient tapestry of Kartikeya and Vali [characters from Indian mythology], which had originally hung in the Murugan Kovil temple in the Sri Lankan village of Kataragama. There was a Shiva trident planted next to a trunk, which our host claimed contained the bones of Adam. Everywhere we looked, we saw symbols and meaning, right down to the base of our coconut bowls that, once drained of liquid, revealed the Kataragama *yantra* [a sacred geometric symbol], which is two interpenetrating triangles forming a six-pointed star.

It occurred to me that I had better be on my best 'spiritual' behaviour! Initially, when people have an interest in spirituality, it is common for them to approach it from an external perspective, and I was no different. I sat there with my spine rod-straight, imagining that I appeared extremely spiritual! I was sitting there, stiff and upright, when Swami Gauribala stopped smack in the middle of a conversation to ask me in a pointed way, 'Why are you sitting like that?' I felt completely disarmed. I had held an attitude that I should appear a certain way in front of such men and he challenged me! I was starting to squirm.

As it happened, an animated debate broke out between our host, Mike Wilson, and the man whom we had come to meet, Swami Gauribala. One would say 'black', the other 'white'. One would say 'all is pure', the other that 'one must purify'. One would say 'yes', the other 'no'. They argued back and forth, intensely and urgently. Being young and in a foreign setting, and feeling overwhelmed by the surrounds and the company, I sat silent and awestruck by the incisiveness of their arguments. Things were starting to get intense, and I was beginning to seriously wonder where this was all going. Suddenly, Mike pinned me down with his eyes and demanded, 'YOU must decide who is God and who is the devil!'

Words failed me. I didn't know what to reply, but I sensed that somehow, perhaps through the force of energy in the room, I had been catapulted into a different state of mind, one that I had never experienced before. Despite being young and quite naive in this world of theirs, I recognised instantly that Gauribala was the man who was going to change my life. An immediate and awesome feeling of love welled up in me for him, such that I had never felt before, and at the same time, this love was mingled with fear. Here was the man who was going to challenge me, teach me. I knew my life would never be the same.

Suddenly, while puffing away on his cigar, Swami asked me intently: 'Who *are* you?' Again and again. It is the classic question of self-enquiry, but of course I didn't know that at the time. 'I'm Rose-Ellen Rockermann,' I answered, relieved that finally I knew the answer to one of his questions. 'Oh, I see,' he replied. 'Yes,' I repeated, 'Rose-Ellen. It's a hyphenated name.' And he continued, 'Oh! You're a hyphen person, are you?' With this comment, I knew that I had missed his point and I was reeling again. 'I am a hyphen person too!' he exclaimed in his jolly tone, and with that he leapt up and dashed into an adjoining room—his energy was amazing, so light on his feet it was as if he didn't touch the ground. Two seconds later he reappeared with a book and the book was entitled *Hyphen People*. And in the book was a chapter on him.

Gauribala was a German who had lived for thirty years in Sri Lanka and had bridged the culture gap so completely that you would mistake him for Tamil—that was what made him, literally, a hyphen person too. It dawned on me that no matter what this man said it was true on many levels. He could make a remark as benign as 'I am a hyphen person', yet he could actually manifest evidence so that what he said became actuality. He spoke always from a place of truth, so that no matter what he said, even through the veiled layers of speech, it became true in every conceivable way: literally and figuratively.

Swami wore only a white *worsti* [sarong] and never shoes; he had a halo of dusty white hair and a beard that flowed to his chest. He wore no rings nor bore any markings, except for a single tattoo on his inner right arm that read *'summa iru'*. A fuming cigar was almost permanently wedged between his lips. On occasion he removed it from his mouth and instead placed it up his nostrils and then in his ears. He huffed and puffed clouds of smoke out of these orifices while rolling his eyes in opposite directions.

Imagine! I was a young seeker earnestly wanting to find a man of wisdom—whom I presumed would be solemn, serious and holy—and what I was confronted by was this kind of craziness. But Swami perceived exactly what my preconceptions of a learned man were: what he should act like, look like, and dress like, and he was challenging me to drop *all* preconceptions. He knew that I was searching for understanding, and he was offering it to me, but first I had to leave behind my textbook ideals and get real. It was in this way that Swami Gauribala continued piece by piece to dismantle, or sometimes to knock down, my preconceptions and conditioning.

Later that night, we left Mike Wilson's home and a small group of us went to dinner, where again Swami pounced on notions I had formed about what it meant to be on the spiritual path. Since I had become this 'spiritual' person living in Maine, naturally I was a pure vegetarian, as I believed that spiritual people should be. And yet when we sat down at the dinner table, meat was served. I was horrified! What I hadn't noticed in myself was that out of my choosing to be vegetarian, a different obstacle had risen up and blinded me. Swami recognised it immediately.

When the meat was passed around, I swiftly handed it on and Swami, who was sitting next to me, cocked an eyebrow and in an exaggerated tone exclaimed: 'Oh! You're a vegetarian. I see!' Again, I was in front of this group I hardly knew, wishing I were anywhere but. 'I am a vegetarian too,' he said, as he helped himself to a serving of goat curry, 'In between meals!!'

These simple but essential teachings were all there. He challenged me outwardly in ways that caused me to become internally transformed. Out of my food preferences, I had developed pride and aversion. I continued to be a vegetarian, but let go of my pride and aversion, and my tendency to judge others based simply on their dietary choices!

As our relationship deepened, I knew that being with Swami was like purification by fire: dangerous and scary, but also quick and thorough. I did not receive teachings in an academic, textbook way. The nature of his lineage is not like this. Rather it was to deliver the teachings in a somewhat 'hidden' way, through silent transmission. Swami's teachings were always imparted in this very immediate, experiential way. This suited me because I am not an intellectual, nor am I a scholar.

One way that a spiritual teacher works is by whittling down the ego that gives us a false sense of ourselves and obscures us from seeing who we truly are. Very early on, I recognised that Gauribala held the sword that was going to chop off my head. He was the one who was going to slay 'Rose-Ellen', to expose my ego for what it was. Of course, ego is necessary to function on this plane—without it you wouldn't eat or care to breathe—but what the guru recognises is the delusional aspect of the ego. The delusional aspect is that which has adopted limiting beliefs about who or what one is and which then constantly projects those limited beliefs outwardly. A person can definitely still work on dissolving the ego without the help of a guru, but the guru accelerates this process. He wields a very sharp sword, while you pound away slowly with a very blunt instrument.

When you sit down with such a teacher, very soon your idea of yourself is going to be rattled to its deepest foundation. because of this that fear is present when you first recognise

the 'assassin'. At the heart level, there is a resonant
connection that allows you to trust this person with the job of
cutting off your head, but rivulets of fear can initially cause
turbulence and doubt. Bravery and courage are required because
you are putting your head on the line. Certainly there were
moments when I wanted to run away spurred on by doubts or
paranoia, but my deepest driving desire to know who I truly
was kept me riveted. However trying my time with Swami
became, I stayed on in order to learn.

I find it difficult to describe Swami's teachings and perhaps
this story will illustrate why. One day my boyfriend and I were
visiting him in Colombo at Mike Wilson's home when our
host's two lovely young daughters came skipping into the room.
They sat down next to Swami who turned to me and asked,
'Can you sing us a song?' It was a simple request but one that
I couldn't fulfil. Instead of breaking into song, I went mute.
I felt drenched in a sudden wave of self-consciousness as I
realised that I couldn't 'just' sing a song. Of course, Swami
wasn't asking me to just sing a song; he was highlighting my
lack of spontaneity, my absence of childlike joyfulness, and a
sense of self-consciousness that had crept up on me over the
years. Instead he turned to the two little girls and asked them,
'Can you sing a song?' And they burst into an adorable little
song. There we were, them singing sweetly and me having a
profound realisation about how I had traded childlike spontaneity
and joyfulness for self-consciousness and posturing.

The girls kept singing away until Swami made a *mudra*
[gesture that alters flow of energy in the body] with his hand
and the two girls froze, mid-tune. They were held in mid-air.
During these moments of suspended animation, I felt as if
Gauribala was transferring volumes of unspoken information.

For this reason it is almost impossible to articulate his teachings: by their very nature, they are secret and sacred. There is no risk that what he taught will be distorted because there is simply nothing to be said. After a few moments he made the *mudra* again and the girls recommenced singing as if nothing had happened. This event took me weeks to digest and assimilate. What I was experiencing seemed to be so far removed from everyday life, but at the same time I sensed that it was somehow intricately connected and woven into it.

As Ramesh Nayak, a Vedic astrologer I had the pleasure of meeting recently, so beautifully commented: 'An artist is one whose absorption in the moment is so absolute that he will make the flute play the flute and then burn it all before the audience. The performance is only the tip of the iceberg— what needs preserving are the hidden factors that created it. This is encompassed in the guru–*shishya* [teacher–disciple] relationship.'

On another occasion, after Swami had left Colombo and returned to the northern town of Jaffna, we decided to visit him in his hermitage. We travelled across Sri Lanka and arrived so wired with anticipation that when he greeted us by showing us where we could lie down and take a nap, I thought, 'I'm too excited to take a nap! There's no way I can sleep now!' Nevertheless, he took us into a hut and instructed, 'Lay down here and I will see you in a little while.' I lay down reluctantly where he pointed and fell asleep instantly—*instantly!* I didn't wake up until the moment he walked back into the room. These were the kinds of inexplicable experiences I was having.

Swami Gauribala was a *sannyasin*, a renunciate, who had spent seven years meditating deep in the hills of Sri Lanka in Ravana's cave [where King Ravana hid Sita after he kidnapped her from Rama, in the epic *Ramayana*]. For many years he walked the Padayatra, a pilgrim's trail that winds and stretches for 350 miles from Jaffna in the north to the sacred village of Kataragama in the south. This itself is a meditation. Over time it started to sink in just what this man had sacrificed and relinquished in order to remain steadfast on his spiritual path. Few in the world are able to put that kind of life energy into their *sadhana*. And just as he could sit in a cave for years and meditate in seclusion, he could also be the life of the party in any mundane situation, because for him there was no separation anywhere whatsoever.

Once I expressed to him my sense of hopelessness that I would ever reach his level of awareness. I could never see myself spending seven years in a cave or walking on red-hot coals. 'You don't have to do anything!' he said and started bubbling, dancing and prancing about, chiming effervescently, 'There's nothing to do in the house of bamboo, but everybody needs a hobby!'

His instruction was always so simple, but it would sustain me like a rock throughout times of crises and doubt. And those times were to come. Whenever I found myself in turmoil, I would recall his simple words. They were potent, becoming like an antidote when I felt poisoned by some afflictive emotion, and at other times as soothing as a sweet lullaby when I felt sad or alone. '*Summa iru*,' he told me, '*Summa iru*. Simply be. Simply be.'

## LEAVING

I reached a point where I wanted to leave Sri Lanka because things were moving too fast for me. Meeting Gauribala had opened an area in my psyche where it appeared that whatever

I desired would manifest itself in the most profound and obvious way—so much so that it started to frighten me. I started to feel paranoid; I felt so vulnerable and open, like my every thought was being exposed. Upon reflection, I can see that I was experiencing the early stages of disintegration of the personality, but at the time I didn't understand what was happening. Only later did I understand that you experience paranoia because your personality is all that you have foolishly known yourself to be—when that starts falling away, there is a period of identity crisis, fear that things will get out of 'your' (ego's) control.

I was twenty-three years old by this time and starting to seriously wish that everything would return to 'normal'. I wanted my life to feel 'safe' and 'within my control' again. My destiny had unfolded according to my desire. I had met the man of wisdom and knowledge who had woken me up. Quickly, skilfully and with exquisite precision, Swami had made me acutely aware of my pride, self-consciousness and the other personality traits that prevented me from realising the truth about who 'I am'. He exposed the *vasanas* [habitual tendencies] and *samskaras* [personality traits] that sustained my ego—but I needed a break. I wanted things to lighten up! In Sri Lanka I left behind the man who threatened to deconstruct the notion of 'Rose-Ellen Rockermann'. Instead I felt deep, powerful, primal instincts urging me towards sex, marriage and motherhood.

These urges were about playing out my *karma* and *rnanubandhanas* [bondage of karmic debt]. My daily life became less mystical and magical and more practical and mundane—well, sort of. Jon Hawley and I had since broken up. I married a man called John Collingwood and settled in India, maintaining a beach house in Goa during the winter and a mountain abode in the Himalayas during the summer. At thirty-one I became pregnant and was blessed with my son, Aaron. I spent more than a decade practising *asana, pranayama* and meditation with various teachers, as well as dancing the night away at full moon parties, all while raising my son on the beach, under the coconut trees, watching the sun sink into the warm waters of the Arabian Sea.

My husband and I travelled extensively throughout India to visit many of the countless sacred temples and holy places, from Ramaswaram on the southern tip to Armanath Cave high in the Himalayas, but at the time I didn't fully understand the esoteric significance of pilgrimage and of what was in front of me. Only years later did I realise that the external pilgrimage is analogous to the inner journey from periphery to centre, from mundane to divine, from temporal to eternal. I was being exposed to the power of ritual over and over again, and as I fostered this devotion and reverence for a spiritual life, so ripened within me a willingness to surrender my will to a higher power.

For twelve years I did not see Swami, but he was permanently enshrined in my heart and mind. I worked through all kinds of gnarly *karma*: material desires, addictions, difficult domestic issues, major relationship challenges concerning sex and money. After one decade of marriage, it was clear that my relationship was in deep trouble. To obtain clarity, I attended a twenty-day silent mediation retreat. The result? Our marriage ended. Leaving Aaron (who was by now five years old) in India with his father with the intention of returning three weeks later, I went to Europe to pursue a very passionate relationship. My lover and I were doing a lot of meditation, *asana, pranayama* and also engaging in intense intimacy—all of which have the tremendous potential to open you up physically, mentally, emotionally, psychically, spiritually—when one morning we were sitting in meditation and I suddenly heard the voice of my guru.

It was as if I was seeing and hearing some sort of hologram of Swami Gauribala that appeared before me, as well as inside me—as if I was on the inside, as well as on the outside. 'You must return to Sri Lanka to close my eyes,' he said, precisely and concisely. I have always had strong intuition, but this was absolutely unlike anything that had ever happened to me before. I was not fantasising, I wasn't sitting there daydreaming and I hadn't dropped off into a doze. I was fully conscious, fully awake and fully aware that what had just occurred was a telepathic communication. Subtle ears received subtle speech. Subtle eyes had seen subtle form. Strong practice may have prepared my psychic receptors, but it was Gauribala who was exhibiting his abilities from afar.

There was no question in my mind of what to do. Without hesitating, the flight was booked and two days later I boarded the plane for Sri Lanka. This was a time of turbulent upheaval and intensity in my life: my marriage had ended, my young son wasn't with me, I was abruptly abandoning my lover, I had received this sober message in a most bizarre fashion, and Sri Lanka was in the middle of a violent and bloody war. I doubted whether Gauribala would even to be in the same place after twelve years. But all those years before, he had taught me the way to cross the most difficult situations—*summa iru*, simply be. Again the power of *summa* carried me forward.

I had to keep reminding myself that I knew why I was going. I had received a message that was real and true. There was no need to think, just to go! I randomly opened up the book I was carrying with me, *Tibetan Yoga and Secret Doctrines* by W.Y. Evans-Wentz, and searching for inspiration I read:

'Do not imagine, do not think, do not analyse. Do not meditate, do not reflect; keep the mind in its natural state.' Good idea! I wondered instead what movie was showing on the flight.

Finally the plane landed at Bandaranike airport and I made my way to Colombo for the night. I thought I would travel to Jaffna by train early the next morning, but the Tamil Tigers had blown up the railway. The raging civil war made it extremely difficult and dangerous to move about, especially to Jaffna, seat of the insurgents. After an exhausting trip in a beaten up old minibus I finally reached my destination. I approached the temple as if in a dream just as Gauribala stepped out and into my sight. I wondered if he would remember me after my long absence. '*Padma!* Rose!' he said after a moment, 'You've come home.' My heart swelled with emotion and tears streamed from my eyes—the whole chain of events had been so incredible. The next three weeks spent with my teacher in his hut became the most significant of my life. I didn't make any mention of the telepathic message that had brought me there. When I first entered his room, he asked me to go to Jaffna to buy some whisky. 'What sort?' I asked. 'TEACHER'S Whisky, of course!' was his reply.

As I said before, Gauribala speaks a 'twilight' language: there is always an unspoken dialogue going on. I felt tremendously privileged to be in his company. He took me to Yogaswami's *samadhi* (his guru's shrine). He instructed me on the four *Mahavakyas* [great truths]. He told me I should have been there ten years ago! I felt regret for running away all those years before.

The good news was that Swami seemed to be in perfect health, and after several weeks I figured that I must have been deluded with my 'vision' in Amsterdam. Although filled with gratitude and deep peace to be in his presence, it was time for me to go back and sort out my life. I had been away from Aaron for nearly a month and was very concerned about him. I had to face the *karmic* wreckage of my actions: divorce, child custody, property settlement. After telling Swami my plans to leave, he said, 'Wait. In three days you will close my eyes.'

Although I had heard those very words one month before, I was stunned. Past, present and future all converged to a single point. Thereafter, all and any doubts that remained about my relationship with Gauribala were annihilated, instantly reduced to cinders. This affirmed our eternal connection, absolutely unconditioned by time or space.

Still, I didn't mention anything to him of the vision I had. I didn't burst out with, 'I know! I saw and heard you say that one month ago!' I was silent. The very next day, Gauribala lay down on his thin straw mat in his hut near the temple in preparation to consciously leave his body behind. I was struck by his offering to me this life-altering gift of exquisite intimacy; this is the grace of the guru.

He displayed calm, focused attention on exactly what was happening and where he was going. 'Are you going to transmigrate [move spirit from one's own body into that of another person]?' I asked, hoping that somehow I would still be able to visit him in physical form. 'No,' he replied, 'but I can choose my womb' [conscious rebirth is a high yogic ideal]. Talk about being prepared for a trip!

For three days, I sat by his mat-side with tender young coconut-water, offering sips when he needed them. On the third day, he was staring straight up without blinking for what seemed like hours. I thought to myself, 'I wonder if he is still conscious?' He flashed his gaze on me with such tremendous

intent and penetrating intensity that I knew I had irritated
by being dense about what I was witnessing: fearless surrender
to the Mother. [The 'Mother' is another name for Creation, a
Tantric euphemism for the life-giving force behind the cosmos.]

Later that day, it became obvious that the life-force had begun
to withdraw from his physical body; the energy in the room was
super-charged. The illusory veil of worldly existence was being
torn away, ripped asunder. On that third day, I indeed closed his
eyes. As I lay next to his body that night, I heard him utter *'Umma'*
[Mother] thrice. He was back in the arms of the beloved Mother.

The next day, the temple priest, Swami Mayilvahanam,
approached and said, 'You were summoned here, so it is you
who must perform the ceremony in preparation for his
cremation.' With their guidance, I did so as if in a very familiar
dream. I was given a bowl of burning camphor and led the
procession to the cremation ground. Swami's body lay atop
the funeral pyre, bedecked with flowers and offerings, as I
circumambulated three times and lit the fire under his head.
The next morning I was requested to perform the ritual over
any remaining bones. They were then gathered and placed on
a tray, which I carried on my head as I walked to the back of
his hut and into the river, waist-deep. As I tipped my head back,
the bones slid into the river, signalling the end of my relationship
with my guru in physical form.

## ENTERING THE INNER TEMPLE

I never considered the notion of initiation until I returned to
Colombo and related all that had happened to those who were
closest to Swami. I met Mahen; for generations his family has

been the temple custodians and landowners of an island off Jaffna where Hanuman [the Monkey god] first landed on his heroic leap to retrieve Sita [kidnapped wife of Rama in the epic *Ramayana*]. 'Make no mistake,' he told me convincingly, 'You have been initiated into the Tantric Siddhas of Tamil Nadu.' I had never heard of them before. For me, the first initiation was Gauribala's symbolic 'cutting off of the head'. Then twelve years of fulfilling desires and burning *karma* had passed before the second initiation: the request to close his eyes and to be present at his death-mat. And again, after Gauribala's *Mahasa-madhi* [conscious exit from the body], I spent another twelve years cooking up and eating my *karma*. I left India and settled in Australia. I entered another marriage. I acquired a beautiful property and a beautiful house. Aaron was healthy, an achiever in school, a kind, quiet and independent child. Despite all this, I was still repeating the same difficult lessons, sabotaging my relationships with habitual patterns and conditioned responses, winding up in similar situations that were pregnant with dissatisfaction. Due to the insistence of my second husband, Marc Baudin, I began teaching yoga in Australia. Several years later, I received an invitation to teach overseas which began a sojourn of teaching in some of the most exotic locations on the planet. Externally, everything looked perfect, but internally the battles were still raging. Considering the fact that I had done so much study and practice of yoga, and in the light of my experiences with my guru, how was it possible that I could still be so stuck? My marriage wasn't working and I divorced again.

I was in Tahiti, where I still teach seminars regularly, and decided to do a personal silent retreat. I felt that I had reached limitations in my understanding of how to proceed with my *sadhana*, and with my life. During that time I supplicated

Gauribala in desperation. 'I need your guidance,' I implored him. I had reached a stagnation point and could see no way to stir that stagnation into activity. A total internal restructuring needed to take place to free me from my self-imposed limitations. I knew what needed to happen, but didn't know how to do it.

For five days I did not move from meditation. I begged and pleaded with my guru to show me how to proceed. 'I don't care if it kills me,' I insisted, 'I am not moving from this spot until you come up with something. It is your responsibility! You are my guru! With or without a body, it makes no difference! Show me the next step!'

I got a response. Swami Gauribala addressed me thus: 'Simply place yourself in the arms of the Mother. What does a baby need to do when cradled in the arms of its mother? Nothing. *Summa iru.*' He had left his body by doing just this, simply surrendering his life-force to Her. I was ecstatic. It is worth mentioning, however, that this instruction could be dangerously misinterpreted—be careful! It is not by simply lying back in the hammock that life will automatically move in the right direction.

After my seminar concluded, I left Tahiti and went back to Australia where another surprise awaited me. On my kitchen table, in a pile of mail, were several special letters. One was from Jon Hawley with whom I had first met Gauribala thirty years earlier. He stated that every night for the past two weeks Gauribala had been in his dreams, in which Swami had breathed an 'unfathomably deep breath' into him.

Hmmmm. Amazing coincidence? Perhaps.

Then I picked up the next letter. It was from Manik Sangras-agra, the man who had initially approached us on the beach in Colombo and told us about Swami. 'Sam Wickramasinghe has just contacted me,' he wrote. 'He has had a dream in which Swami has appeared with a message for you.' I couldn't believe what I was reading.

These two letters, back-to-back with my experience in silent retreat, catapulted me into space that knows no boundaries. There was a shift of consciousness. I fell into a psychic corridor that re-established my contact with the *parampara* of my guru [connection to the guru's lineage is like being invisibly linked to an immediate body of teaching and spiritual awareness].

I had never heard of this Sam before, and was intrigued by the involvement of a new 'character' in the play. I contacted him as soon as I could—though it took some time to get his telephone number. I discovered that in the fifties Sam had met Gauribala in the jungle shrine of Kataragama and later spent some years with him and Yogaswami in Jaffna. He told me that he was supposed to give me information that Gauribala had not had time to give me.

He could not do this over the phone and told me that I would have to go to Sri Lanka to sit with him so that it would be absolutely clear what he was giving me. There could be no room for misinterpretation. I asked him when I should come. His answer was: 'You have to look into your own heart for that. Meanwhile, I will send you a letter with the message from the dream.' I awaited this letter with the anticipation of a lover waiting for news of the beloved.

Several weeks later I received the message from Sam's dream that represented the third initiation:

Tell her to seek the *padma* (lotus) in the *guha* (cave) of her sacred heart. Wherein one could experience the mystery of *summa*, the eternal presence and the mystique of the now, which is, always is, unconditioned by time or space, or any other contingency of life.

A few months later I met with Sam at his home in Minuwangoda, where he shared his knowledge of Tantra with me and, well, that's a whole other story. After this last 'initiation' I am working out a different kind of *karma*. It appears that many of my old patterns have truly dried up and blown away, yet some still remain. Different challenges arise, but I welcome the opportunity to manipulate the energy of potentially 'difficult' situations and use it as fuel for my *sadhana*. As Gauribala used to say, 'The worse, the better!'

Staying aware of the direction in which you are heading requires keen observation of *citta nadi* [the mindstream]. When you expose what is in the mindstream, then you can understand where that current is taking you. Is it towards Reality [the Self] or towards delusion or ignorance [*avidya*]? When you jump into the ocean, it's smart to check out the current lest you get carried away in a rip! To keep your awareness [*nivritti eye*] fixed on your breath as passionately as a nursing babe regards its mother is to step onto the magic carpet.

Staying focused and cultivating devotion to Reality is a challenge! Cultivating the concentration to maintain the perpetual inner practice of non-attachment is a challenge! It's is so easy to fall short; we are not always honest with ourselves about what it is we really want—and as it says in the *Upanishads* what we want we will eventually get. This is how our *karmas* pile up, and we spend many, many lifetimes trying to burn up those afterwards.

Swami Gauribala was an accomplished human being. It was as if he was absolutely transparent, casting no shadow, letting the light pass through him to illuminate everything around him. Although a renunciate, he could operate with as much ease in the mundane world with others as he could meditating in solitude in the cave.

As it said in the letter, the yogic path is about discovering the inner temple. Gauribala has been my teacher, my guru, and my beloved mentor. He is the man of wisdom whom I desired to meet when I was very young and he has guided me deftly on my path. He revealed the extraordinary in the ordinary and the divine in the mundane. He taught me that if it is not here, it is nowhere. To reside in the ecstasy of the inner temple is the essence of *summa iru*.

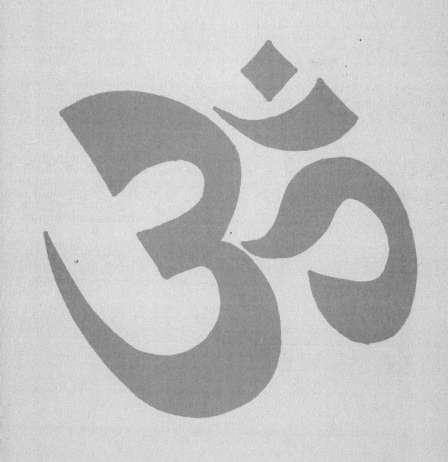

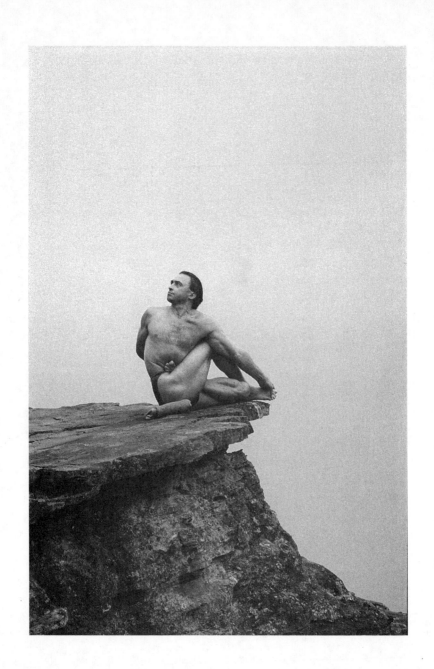

# 7

# MOVING INTO THE LIGHT

## *Shandor Remete*

*The nervousness! Don't perform for me. The unease that one feels is not for me, it is for one's Self. It is okay to make mistakes.*

Shandor Remete

At age six the young Hungarian, Shandor Remete, began to practise yoga. In his late twenties he visited India and first studied with his teacher, B.K.S. Iyengar. In his thirties he became one of the most revered and feared teachers outside of India. Yoga Journal called him a 'maverick on the mat' and a 'rock star in tights'. Some call him a true adept whose authority is hard earned. Others: a brute, a hotshot, a terror. His name is an enigma, his practice and teaching are both characterised by ferocity and fervour. At forty-two he was at the peak of his abilities but all that was to change. Soon, things fell apart.

In quick succession his wrist broke, his marriage ended, his father died. He gained weight, no matter how little food he consumed. The Hatha yogi who had spent years cultivating a sublime asana practice could no longer muster the energy to do even the simplest poses. The yoga Remete thought would safeguard him from injury and disappointment failed him. Reeling, he stood back and asked the question: What went wrong?

Remete could not in good faith continue to practise and teach as he had before—and yet he could not walk away either. Yoga was his life's work. Instead, he assumed a beginner's mind. He returned to the source: consulting ancient Sanskrit texts and seeking out Indian masters from whom he would relearn yoga. This time he searched with eyes wide open and became watchful, filling in the gaps that he had overlooked before. This about-face revealed a vulnerability previously concealed beneath the armour of success.

Now in his mid-fifties, Remete is still a formidable figure. Despite the deep lines on his beautiful face, the greying shorn hair and the hooded eyes, his body remains taut, muscular and lean, his tongue sharp and his charisma bright. Although famous, he is not proud of yoga's current popularity and status in the media spotlight. He says that when all the 'hype' blows over, only the dedicated and the sincere will remain.

Since his epiphany, Remete no longer teaches Hatha yoga in the Iyengar style but in his own style, Shadow yoga [Chaya Samyukta]. Outwardly, it is different, he says, but the intent remains the same: to go beyond the shadows—who we think we are—and return to the source, the light—who we truly are.

Just as his career has been unconventional, and to some controversial, this is, he might say, just the shadow that masks the inner person. It is twilight by the time Remete finishes his practice, as he began it two hours earlier, seated in padmasana [lotus]. One pose flows seamlessly into the next, his body bends and opens gracefully, fluidly, while his eyes look somewhere else unseen, perhaps to the world within. His body glows faintly from the effort and is backlit by the afternoon sun as it makes its descent into night. He twines his legs together, slips right foot over left hip and left foot over right, lets his knees rest lightly on the ground and brings his hands to touch, finger to finger, palm to palm, in front of his chest. He completes his practice, head bowed, in silent meditation. This practice is an art form worthy of an audience, but on this afternoon, it is just Remete and a few others milling around the studio. An afternoon like any other. His practice over for the day, Remete, one of the western world's brightest teaching lights, talks about the development of Shadow yoga.

## OPEN YOUR EYES

Yoga is the reverse process of life. If life takes one outwards and away from the source of one's Self, then yoga is the path back in. Even this path is not foolproof. I made mistakes and

I have spent the last twelve years undoing the mistakes I began making when I was six.

I was born into a family where my father was already doing yoga. He would practise *asana*, *mudra* and *bandha* behind a closed door and I would wonder what he was doing. One day I looked in and started mimicking what I saw. He supported that monkeying around and that is how I learnt. By six I was doing basic seated poses and inversions. *Yogasana* [another word for *asana*] was never imposed on me, I chose to investigate it out of my own curiosity. Being born into a family where yoga was practised was both a blessing and a curse. I say curse because it was my familiarity with it that would lead me to overlook the basic forms and cause me to make mistakes.

I grew up in Northern Yugoslavia until I was about seventeen years old. At school I studied gymnastics and speed skating. When my family moved to Australia, I began studying martial arts too. I served in South Vietnam and afterwards I found B.K.S. Iyengar's book, *Light On Yoga*, and began practising all these poses that I didn't know existed. I went to India where I studied with Iyengar.

It was never my intention to teach yoga, things just evolved. I used to practise *yogasana* every day and one day a friend who had seen me practise asked me to teach him how to do the poses. I refused, but said he could practise alongside me. He agreed, knowing that I would not be able to tolerate any sloppiness of style, and before long I was off my mat and busy correcting him. That is how I started teaching. Within a week my small house was filled with students.

In the early days students paid me by donation. I left an honesty box by the front door and they would leave a few dollars. That system stopped the day I caught a guy putting three bucks in and taking twenty out! Next I established schools in Adelaide, Melbourne and Sydney and began to take on apprentices. Over time, invitations started to come to travel overseas and teach and before I knew it, I had fallen into another thing. Naturally, as things evolve, you hope to be good at what you do, but in wanting to be good at what you do you project from your ego self and you end up making a lot of mistakes. And if you have a lot of fire in you, like I do, partly by virtue of my Hungarian blood, you leave a trail of enemies. But even that slowly educates you. All these events unfolded and my life evolved like this because I had chosen to follow a driving intent, to follow a path that I had chosen for myself, which is to know and meet the source of all things.

One thing led me to another, then that evolved into something else, and so on. I know that nothing lasts forever. And at each stage in my life, there has been reflection, and at each crossing over into the next phase, you change. Will this lead to an ultimate destination? I think that paths are just paths. One path leads here and the next leads there. All along the way there are junctions and when you reach a junction you make a decision. This is how my life has unfolded.

I have now reached a point where I don't care what the world thinks of me anymore. That people benefit from what I do is good, but fame is just a by-product. Everyone wants to be famous—famous this, famous that—what for? I know now that when my activities are harmonious with the way the world is, when they project not what is personal but what is necessary, only then can I walk away with the fulfilment of the experience of life itself. And that is enough. In other words, it is enough to be a human being, and yoga is a system that enables you to become a better human being.

Many people doing yoga are as lost as they were before they began. People think yoga is about how great a backbend or forward bend one can do, or even how flexible one is. It is not. Yoga is about cultivation of the spirit and cultivation of the individual. When the spirit is strong and steady, then the yoga practice is good. You can be as flexible as you like and do as many postures as possible but if the intellect is weak, if there is no emotional stability, then this is not a true yoga practice. In this way the practice of *yogasanas, pranayama* and meditative states are nothing but tools in one's hands that can be used to maintain a level of inner stability. They are meant to bring about an understanding of one's Self. Only then is one able to relate *to* the world, and *within* the world, in a balanced and harmonious manner. Only then will one not be disturbed by the events of life, but will be able to adapt and respond to any situation that arises. It is important to understand these tools well, because if you do not understand the tools in your hands, then you are not a skilful person. And when you are not skilful, you can end up making many mistakes.

I made mistakes because of my familiarity with the subject. Because I started yoga at age six, and because I was physically able, I did not understand the need for the basic forms as I do now. Could my teacher have prevented this? The role of the teacher is to point the student in a certain direction that they might follow, but if I am at fault, it is of my own doing.

My father was my first teacher of Hatha yoga, but I have had many other teachers in life. I think all teachers that you connect with contribute to your journey; my mathematics teacher and my language teachers contributed just as much to my self-growth as any other teacher who has helped to open up avenues inside me. Of course, the teacher who influenced me most was B.K.S. Iyengar himself. I went to India in the late seventies and began studying with him. Last year someone asked me how the Shadow yoga I now teach fits in with Iyengar yoga. I said, 'If you don't see it, then I am not going to tell you! Nothing but what I have learnt from Iyengar has brought me to this point!' I still recall all the basic principles I learnt with Iyengar, they are still in me, and what I teach is still grounded in them. It is just that they are dressed up differently.

Let me put it another way: you learn many things in life, but you never use them the way you learnt them. At school you learnt mathematics, but when you go out into the world you have to use the rules you learnt according to the situation— shopping, for instance—and it becomes different to how it was presented in the classroom. If you cannot use those rules in the real world, then really you learnt nothing. In the same way, I have applied the yoga learnt with various teachers to my own life.

It is true that I saw some things that I was unhappy with in the yoga I was practising: unhappy because they were not bearing results. I was repeating things that were totally useless and I was aware that they were useless. So what do you do when you come across something that is lacking in meaning to you? You have to examine it. When you realise something is lacking, it doesn't matter anymore who is who or what is what, you have to look for the honest truth inside yourself and then ask yourself this: Are you following something with blind faith, or are you walking around with open and observing eyes? There is a huge difference.

Yoga is not about blind faith. You must have faith in your own personal undertaking and know that you are learning—

otherwise you are just a projection of your own mind—you are not moving beyond the shadows, but getting tangled in them. I find people are often threatened by a practice that is different from their own. They shouldn't be. Instead, they should look with open eyes at what is new and what is familiar about the practice. In yoga there is sometimes a tunnel-vision approach where practitioners declare that 'my style is better than yours'. Styles are just styles. The different styles of yoga are beneficial for promoting different things. They each have a plus and a minus.

## SEEING THROUGH BLIND FAITH

About twelve years ago I was faced with a number of losses. I used to practise yoga for ten hours a day: physically I was able, it was all there. And then for the first time ever, my capacity was gone. At the same time my father died. My marriage ended. I broke my wrist. All of a sudden my body blew up. I was doing all this practice, ten hours a day, and I was becoming heavier and heavier. I had to eat, so I ate one meal a day. Still, I continued to blow up like a balloon. 'Excuse me,' I said, 'what is this?' I was doing everything that the experts said to do and nothing helped. I could not use my body. I tried the simplest of positions and I would pass out for two hours. Nobody could give me an answer.

From that crisis, I decided that I would have to go back to point zero to investigate what was going on. So I went back and I stood outside my world and began to see it with new eyes. I studied martial arts again, this time with the Shaolin temple monks. I studied with a Japanese sword master who was ninety-four years old, with the traditional dancers of South India and in non-commercial yoga schools in India, and I started to see where things went wrong with the yoga. Slowly, I started to realise that what needed to be taught was how to observe your own behaviour towards yourself.

In my search I encountered a very interesting interpretation of the *Hatha Yoga Pradipika* by Swatmarana, author of one of the most important texts on Hatha yoga from the fourteenth century. What was interesting is that the *Hatha Yoga Pradipika* usually has four chapters only, yet the text that I came across had five. The fifth chapter speaks about therapy. The first *sloka* [Sanskrit verse] of this additional chapter lists the number of diseases that can result from erroneous practice of *asana* and *pranayama*. What was important to memorise from this lost chapter was that you cannot just do *asana* any which way, you cannot place blind faith in the belief that because you are doing yoga you will arrive here or there, because you may in fact be opening yourself up to disease. Instead, you must investigate it appropriately, and slowly apply yourself with the help of a guide. Of course, who wants to investigate slowly and do only what a guide tells you to do?

In today's big yoga hype, people want to do all the advanced poses first. But if you look at the average person who comes to a yoga class today, they are too stiff to do even the most basic of the forward bend positions—*janu sirsasana* can be extremely difficult for the average beginner and can cause problems. *Trikonasana* [standing triangle pose] can be very difficult too. So there needs to be something that brings beginners to that place. The answer is that you have to start with poses that closely resemble basic daily activities: standing, squatting, walking and lunging. To a certain extent these everyday activities are lost on the individual in the modern world. Those activities of standing, squatting, sitting and lunging develop the intuitive qualities of the body. They awaken intuitive intelligence. They develop consciousness and conscious behaviour. When your understanding is subtle enough to comprehend the actions and functions of the different body parts, then you are able to function intelligently without going against the body's natural energy structures.

This is what has been left out of yoga today: developing the intuitive intelligence of the body, which is very different from projected intelligence. Intuitive intelligence develops conscious behaviour, not projected behaviour.

In India, daily life includes these basic bodily positions, so the need for preparatory work is not so crucial. Still, if you go to the non-commercial yoga schools, which are little and few, the preparatory work has not been left out. These teachers are not interested in you coming and going as you please, either you get involved and you move slowly through the process of learning, or they are not going to teach you at all. It is as simple as that.

What I found amazing is that the preparatory movements that train beginners for internal arts like the dance and martial arts of South India, Northern India, China and Japan are the same movements that prepare one for yoga. In South India, the martial artists are massaged daily for up to three months and are then put into a steam or sweat to make the soft tissues responsive. Once the soft tissues are responsive, they are put into training. For two to three years all they do is basic, very simple, training. Once the basics are learnt properly, the body will open up and the advanced poses will come.

Shadow yoga grew out of the field of my activities and it

sums up the understanding that I have of yoga. It took me many years to investigate the principals that I have incorporated. The information is very sparse in all the Sanskrit texts, but there are clues. I had to investigate in the appropriate places to find the information. I heard my guru mention the *marmashastra* [the study of vital trigger points of energy on the body] and so I investigated. The texts talk about the *vayus* [currents of energy in the body], the *chakras* [major energy centres in the body], the *nadis* [subtle energy pathways] and all of this information had to be integrated intelligently into a practice. If the practice is correct, energy, *prana*, will flow through the core and the periphery. If the practice is incorrect it can be dangerous. What I do now in my teaching and practice is a prelude to the practice of *asanas*.

## ADDRESSING THE INNER PERSON

Cultivation of the individual can take place on many levels, but what yoga deals with primarily is the inner person. It is a practice that enables the inner person to become and remain stable, so that they may perceive all that surrounds them without being disturbed by what they see. For instance, if you worry what other people think of you, then there is no stability.

There are four enemies in life that man must overcome. The first one is fear, the second one is clarity, the third one is power and the fourth one is the one you cannot do anything about: old age.

In the beginning you are very fearful, there is fear in all of us, and you have to understand that really there is nothing to fear. The only thing that accompanies your time here is death and death is with you every second. People worry about death and yet death is leaving them alone. Why think about dying? The very presence of life shows that you are not dying. When people overcome this fear, it is due to the recognition that there is nothing to fear. This brings clarity.

Clarity can render you full of pride. You buy into the illusion that you are a very important person because you see things clearly, and in that very belief, you lose yourself. Life is not about being important. When you overcome that belief, then you access real power—the power of helping people, the power of union, the power of seeing. But then one takes a stance of arrogance—it kind of comes with the stage—and until one overcomes that arrogance, one pays a price.

Eventually, you overcome these three enemies, but the fourth one, old age, you cannot defeat. Old age limits your experience. Old age will come, even for a Hatha yogi, and you must adapt. Why get attached to youth? Life is what it is.

When I talk about these four enemies, I am not suggesting that an adversary is necessarily a bad thing. You can overcome the first three adversaries in order to prolong the last. The more you can prolong life, the richer it will be, and you can choose to have certain experiences for yourself. You can enter as many paths as you choose. The paths that are the best are the ones that bring you joy.

In this way yoga serves men in the modern world the same way it served those in the ancient world. These worlds are different in appearance, but the same basic principles still govern them. All that goes on around us is a reflection of the collective consciousness. If you manage to draw your focus inward, and if you manage to go past all the shadows [ego projections and worldly illusions], then you will touch some part of you that is pure and truthful. And when you touch that deep source, all outer agendas of how you should be in the world are stripped away.

The texts say that you have three bodies: the gross body, the subtle body and the causal body. The intuitive processes are hidden in the causal body; in our language today, we call that 'the soul'. Everything else shines forth from that—the subtle body is the bridge from the most gross (physical) to the subtle (soul). So the education of the person must begin on the surface. The texts also say that the body is light but is encased in shadow.

Everything is a shadow—you have outside shadows and inside shadows. Your body is composed of the five layers [*koshas*]—what they call the food cover [*annamayakosha*], the lifeforce body [*pranamayakosha*], the mundane activity of the mind [*manomayakosha*], the higher intelligence [*vinjamayakosha*] and then, of course the bliss cover [*anandamayakosha*]—that are interwoven through the three bodies [gross, subtle, causal] as if threaded through a multidimensional web. To work through the web is to work with understanding. We must start from the outside, from the shadow, and move towards the light.

It is said that the outer body is nothing but the shadow of a subtler dimension. In the beginning of time, there was only thought. The vibration of thought was all that existed until it was disrupted by light. And with light came the shadow. When light is cast upon an object, a shadow necessarily falls—shadow is the last bastion of light. The mind is the shadow principle. Everything is a projection of the mind.

You must enquire into these things and you need a good guide. It is the guide who must know how to direct a beginner and then, when the individual is ready, should give them more information. If too much information is given before the student is ready, it will obstruct their learning and cause a kind of spiritual constipation. So, first things first. First, the beginner must have a practical outline. Then this outline gives the student a structure onto which more information can be built. Until then, they rely on the guide and their guidance. Later on, more information is imparted and then slowly the student reclaims responsibility for himself or herself. That is how the *guru–chela* relationship has always been and how it should be. Unfortunately teaching is not always like this these days.

In the west right now, knowledge of yoga is often not being imparted slowly and with care. This is what I find: as something gains popularity, only one aspect of it becomes really popular and that is usually the aspect that can be grasped readily by most people. In the case of yoga it is *asana*, because of the west's familiarity with the physical. But even the physical dimension of yoga is only partially presented—the slow and gradual preparatory aspect has been omitted—and the blame has to be taken by those propagators of yoga who brought it to the west in the beginning. They need to take that responsibility. I know that these are strong words I use, but if you look at yoga today, it is misrepresented—whether it is Iyengar or *ashtanga* or whatever. The poor person who walks into the yoga class has done nothing but sit in front of a computer all day. As I have said, for these people even *trikonasana* or *janu sirsasana* is too much for their body's tissues. They have no stamina, no toning of the muscular-skeletal system, and they have no joint function. If you take them straight into *asana* practice, not much comes of it because they are not ready for it. If their tissues are not responsive and you do a certain action that they are not able to respond to then that action becomes an injury. And the first *yama* that Patanjali gives in the *Yoga Sutras* is 'non-injury'.

Not only are there preparatory stages before people should be taken to *asana*, there are preparatory *sutras* before Patanjali even introduces the concept of *asana*. It is not until after Patanjali has explained the attitude and ethics that yoga requires that he explains what *asana* is ['*sthira sukham asanam*', yoga posture is steady and easy (II:46)]. In the *Yoga Sutras*, Patanjali talks of the eight limbs of self-growth, though most teachers today suggest only part of—*part of!*—one limb. The practice of *asana* has been brought down to the same level of intelligence as any other physical activity happening today. It has been dragged down. Unless the principles, as set out in the ancient texts, are followed then the outlook for yoga is not very good.

Most people today who are doing yoga are very unstable, physically and emotionally. They are also dying of the same illnesses as people who spend most of their time in the pubs. So what is the difference if one does yoga or goes to the pub? What is the purpose of doing yoga if I die from the same disease as my neighbour who has never done yoga in his life?

Two of the oldest yoga texts, the *Vashishtha-Samhita* and the *Yoga-Yajnavalkya*, give nine and eight essential *asanas* respectively. Out of those eight *asanas* mentioned in the *Yoga-Yajnavalkya*, seven are seated postures and one is the balancing posture on the elbows. These really are *asanas* in the truest sense in that they deal with sitting poses; the word *asana* refers to 'a seat' where effort has ceased. The standing poses should be referred to as 'bodily placements', or *sthanas*, which means 'that which is fixed'. Inversions are more a form of *mudra*, or gestures of energetic attentiveness.

When you read the texts, they all assume that before one

enters *asana*, the internal energetic principles and power structures of the body have been grasped physically and intellectually. For example, when you bend your index finger, that is moving energy. What happens to the palm also affects what goes on in the lungs and in the heart.

What has been left out of yoga today has been left out because of the big hype. Hype stimulates people, they get energised and they think they have seen God. Yet when a person is taken slowly through the process and only given information and practices when they are ready, it is a different story. This is called cultivation. If it is not done, a person will have difficulties. If it is done properly, if you investigate yoga appropriately and then slowly apply yourself with a guide, then you will eventually get there.

To sum up what happened to yoga in one word: confusion. You must start to make some studies to understand what this activity is based in and where you want to go with it. That is different from placing blind faith in it. Even if one were to follow the activities I teach, they will gain some understanding—but real understanding must be derived from one's own activity and direct experience. Learning of this nature is personal and cannot be explained in words. Words fall short and others get confused. Yoga is like this.

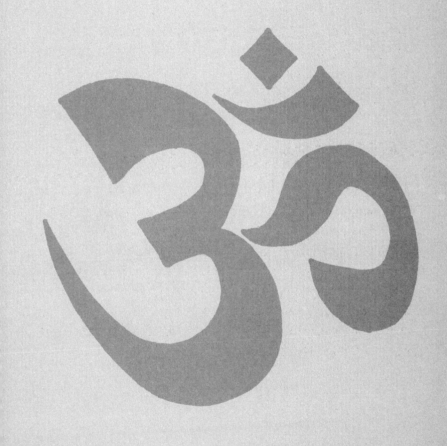

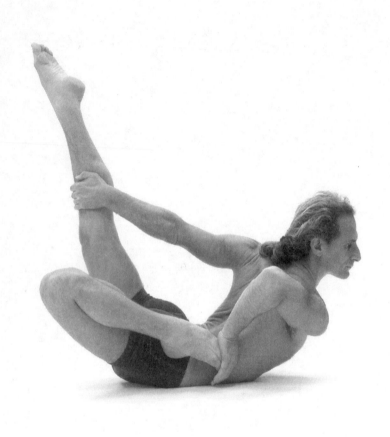

# 8

# HARNESSING ENERGY

## *Simon Borg-Olivier*

*Health, a light body, freedom from cravings, a glowing skin, sonorous voice, fragrance of body: these signs indicate progress in the practice of meditation.*

Shvetashvatara Upanishad

*After class, teacher Simon Borg-Olivier stands by the door of one of his Sydney-based Yoga Synergy schools, and individually farewells almost every student, clasping them by the hand, enquiring, 'How is your partner? Is the knee okay? Thank you for coming.' As his classes brim with over fifty students, this ritual takes some time but he has done it class after class since he began teaching twenty years ago. This simple gesture reveals something of Simon's empathetic nature and also of his approach to yoga: he likes to get involved.*

*According to the dynamic forty-three-year-old, who lives mainly on a diet of raw food and on four hours sleep a night, it was a life-threatening health crisis in his early twenties that forced him to rethink his attitude to his body and that ultimately led him to yoga. Soon yoga became his life's passion.*

*Simon completed a science degree in molecular biology and genetic engineering before making numerous trips to India to study yoga with the great modern masters: B.K.S. Iyengar and the Iyengar family, K. Pattabhi Jois and T.K.V. Desikachar. But a gap appeared: his western body didn't always benefit from how he was practising the eastern techniques of* asana *and* pranayama.

*He returned to university with his business partner and yoga teacher, Bianca Machliss, to study physiotherapy and exercise physiology. Since then, Simon and Bianca have been synthesising what they learnt in the east and the west and have developed a new approach to* asana *that is tailored to suit the western body's needs. Their school, Yoga Synergy, which teaches Synergy-style yoga, attracts around one thousand students each week, accepts five teacher trainees each year, and has offered a course in* Applied Anatomy and Physiology of Hatha Yoga *annually for the past ten years. Simon and Bianca are the co-authors of* Applied Anatomy and Physiology to Hatha Yoga, *a textbook that explains the physiological effects of yoga on the body.*

*Simon's abundance of energy is his trademark and he believes the* ability to harness energy is at the core of yoga practices. He moves like quicksilver around the classroom, trailed by a blur of grey curls. His speech bubbles with warmth and enthusiasm and he is effusive about yoga, dropping to the floor to demonstrate a pose, any pose, mid-conversation. For all the outrageous and wonderful positions into which Simon is able to manipulate his body, he says that, energy aside, what the practice of yoga brings him is mental clarity and peace of mind. There is calm at the centre of the whirlwind of activity.

Our conversation takes place after early morning class and Simon 'drinks' breakfast: one whole rockmelon freshly juiced. He resembles an archetypal yogi: his hair wild and wispy, his chest tanned and toned, his body compact. His voice is mellow and affable. He talks about how it was a lack of vitality that initially brought him to yoga and about what yoga has brought to him.

## YOGA: A MODEL FOR LIFE

I strive for a balance in my life between being a technically minded, intellectually oriented scientist and someone who enjoys a free-form existence and intuitive movement. Yoga enables me to fulfil both. It is a science, an experiment that we conduct with our minds and our bodies, but it is also an exploration of being alive and enjoying life fully. I love what I do—I live it, I eat it, I breathe it—and the ultimate reward for me is being able to share this information with others in a manner that gives me a sense of purpose on the earth.

It is true that the goal of yoga is Self-realisation; however, incorporated into this is being able to enjoy life as much as possible, which in turn involves being able to create as much enjoyment around oneself as possible. I could probably achieve more yogically if I went and fasted on a hillside in solitude, but the word *yoga* itself means union, and that means coming together, not only with yourself but also with other people.

Students and friends sometimes comment that I am a very gregarious, 'out there', on-the-go person. And while I do engage myself in life with many different things at once, I try to do so with mindfulness. Practising the postures and sitting in meditation is time for 'me'. I might be practising in the centre of a classroom, or outdoors in a very public space like a beach or a park, but I am focused, be it on the breath, a gaze point or the sensations in my fingers and toes. This is what Patanjali calls the *dharana* mind, an undisturbed inner focus that generates a sense of clarity and calm. I have tried to take this into all aspects of my day, from working on my Master of Science degree twenty years ago, to being with my wife today. It sounds almost simplistic but this is one of the main reasons I practise yoga: it gives me peace of mind.

The practice of physical postures, *asana*, can be viewed as learning to stay calm and focused under pressure. That's what *asanas* are: artificially induced stressful situations. When you learn to cope under these circumstances—balancing on one leg or upside down on one hand and remaining calm and still in body, breath and mind—then you are better prepared for life, which brings with it stressors that are not so artificially induced. This is how yoga becomes a model for life. *Asana* and *pranayama* improve your fitness and vitality. The *yamas* and *niyamas*, two of the eight limbs of yoga that Patanjali describes in *Yoga Sutras*, cultivate mindfulness, while the meditative states of *pratyahara*, *dharana*, *dhyana* and *samadhi* increase mental fortitude and emotional harmony. In this way the practice of yoga is a means to enhance all aspects of life and, ideally, eventually it also becomes a way of life.

I first began to practise yoga in earnest by applying it to everyday life was when I was doing my Master of Science degree from 1981. It was a very stressful time in my life: I was investigating gene cloning, juggling everyday work, and also beginning to teach yoga. But it was exactly because of the practices of posture, breathing and meditative bliss that I had time and space for regeneration and reflection. My university supervisor, Keith Brown, became one of my best yoga teachers (although he would not see himself that way) because he taught me how to concentrate, how to sustain my focus and not go off the point. This is *dharana* [one-pointed mind]. In a sense all the disparate aspects of my life seemed to join and it felt like I was doing a yoga posture even when I was in the lab conducting an experiment.

What initially brought me to yoga was a need not so much for mental clarity as for physical healing. In my early twenties I experienced an intense healing crisis that changed my life. After completing my undergraduate degree, I began teaching biology practicals to medical students. One day I was in the laboratory teaching and the next I knew I woke up in bed. I had collapsed and some students had carried me to my room. I quickly realised that there was something wrong with my health and that I needed to do something about it.

As a teenager, I didn't care about diet, exercise or what went into my body. I even smoked. After twenty-odd years of chronic abuse, my body couldn't cope and it shut down. I visited a string of doctors who told me that I had the beginnings of all sorts of internal problems. The doctors prescribed a barium enema and medication, and recommended I undergo investigative surgery. I felt sceptical of this drastic treatment and because I was teaching biology to future doctors at the time I (madly) thought that I was just as qualified to heal myself! I took my convalescence into my own hands. After much personal experimentation with so-called cleansing diets I managed to get myself even sicker for a few months! Eventually, however, I became well again; in fact, I would say I reached a euphoric state of health and vitality that I had never felt before, and it was all due to diet, breath and yoga.

This experience taught me one of the most fundamental principles of yoga—*ahimsa* [non-violence]. If you treat your body in a harmful or aggressive way, you will pay a big price. The *yamas* and *niyamas* that Patanjali outlines in the *Yoga Sutras* establish a solid framework for yoga practice, but also for life. I found out very quickly that if it is not good to be aggressive with my body in yoga, then it doesn't pay to be aggressive with my life either.

## YOGA IS ABOUT ATTITUDE

The attitude one has when practising yoga forms the fundamental difference between yoga and conventional forms of exercise. *Yama* and *niyama*, the first and second of the eight limbs of yoga, hold the key to fulfilment in one's life. Non-violence, truthfulness, continence, non-stealing and non-covetousness are learnt on the simplest level in one's practice (these constitute *yama*). Practising without aggression, with an honest recognition of your limitations and with a non-competitive attitude, brings about inner calm instead of frustration, jealousy or injury. On the other hand, *niyama*—especially *tapas* [fervour], *svadhyaya*

[self-study] and *Ishvara pranidhana*, which is com
interpreted as devotion to a higher consciousness but v
see more as a love for everything around us—encourages one
to strive in one's efforts to constantly improve oneself, body
and mind, instead of being complacent.

Bianca and I and the teachers at Yoga Synergy try to bring
these principles into the classroom in subtle but present ways.
For example, we give students the option to work harder or
easier. We give different variations of poses that students can
do according to their body's limitations—for instance, if upward
facing dog is too hard on the wrists we get them to lie on their
tummy and lift their hands and chest. We encourage them to
practise in a non-competitive way and to listen to their body
from breath-to-breath and day-to-day; the poses that suited
someone yesterday might not be appropriate today. This gives
all students the chance to work to capacity, within the boundaries
of non-violence, honesty and non-competitiveness.

As a general rule we find that the *yamas* (such as *ahimsa*,
non-violence) help to soften and restrain the A-type personalities
who want to push themselves no matter what, while the *niyamas*
such as *tapas* [fervour] encourage the B-type personalities to
work a little harder when they might be happy to languish a
little in their practice. Either inclination won't go far without
the counteraction and balancing effect that the philosophy of
yoga offers. Non-aggression with fervour is the ideal approach
to daily practice, as it is a good approach to life.

Yoga is such that the practice teaches you the ethical disciplines without you having to actually pick up a copy of the
*Yoga Sutras* and study them. Ultimately what you learn through
the practice infiltrates everyday life. Someone once said that
the only things you really understand when you read a

philosophical book are the things you already know. When I first read about the *yamas* and *niyamas* I thought I understood them, but it wasn't until I experienced them with my body in my practice that I learnt how wise they really are and how indispensable they are in structuring a sound attitude to life.

To live like this in life at large is to attempt to turn your back on jealousy and to be content with what you have. A lot of life's struggles come from jealousy. Some things in life aren't meant to be yours so why be jealous? One of the biggest liberations for me was honestly acknowledging to myself that some postures were not attainable for me in this body. I had been frustrated by that previously. If you can see what life has given you and be content with that then you will be happier.

I tend more to the A-type end of the personality spectrum and this helped bring me to yoga. After I left school I went to university. After completing my first degree I decided to do another, but I figured that I should also try getting active or else I would end up totally immobilised by stiffness. It was the early eighties and aerobics was big. I like to do anything I take on to the full and soon I was going to aerobics classes twice a day between lectures and tutorials. In my over-zealousness I managed to get shin splints, knee injuries and back problems. I tried other sports. Fencing I enjoyed, although at my first competition I got overexcited and did my best impersonation of Errol Flynn, at which my opponent got very excited back and pierced the skin of my arm. In *tae kwon do* I did my first high kick with so much gusto that I 'dislocated' my buttock. And at gymnastics class I attempted my first backflip and landed on my head, suffering a crush fracture at C5, which to this day means that my neck is very stiff. (My neck was a problem anyway because I have an inflammatory condition called Scheuermann's disease that causes rigidity of the spine.) All these issues brought with them an upside: I had things to fix.

After two years of aerobics the star jumps just weren't happening anymore! My knees were badly damaged and I had ongoing shin splints. I complained to my aerobics instructor and she gave me an exercise that was in fact *supta virasana* [lying back between bent knees]. Almost straight away my shin splints and knees began to get better. I asked for more exercises and she told me to come to her yoga class.

I went along and enjoyed it very much, and then one day a new teacher took over. She was an Iyengar-style yoga instructor and I was awed by what she knew. Initially I was the stiffest person in the room. I sat in *baddha konasana* [feet together knees wide] with my kneecaps up around my ears. In *upavishta konasana* [legs wide forward bend] my fingertips couldn't touch my calves. Aerobics had made me strong and cardiovascularly fit, and I could hold my breath for a long time because my father had taught me how when I was young and learning to swim underwater, but flexibility was not part of my repertoire.

This was around the time that I began to suffer the effects of chronic abuse of the body and realised that I had to address my health. I decided to treat myself and, as I mentioned, nothing worked until, in a final attempt to heal my body, I put myself on a series of fasts. I spent three weeks in silent personal retreat, fasting on spring water in an old volcanic crater in northern New South Wales. Following that I spent six months alternating between two weeks of vegetable juices and two days of salads. At the end of this series of fasts I had a massive clearing from my system that left me feeling completely clean. At the same time my yoga practice changed almost overnight. I went from being the stiffest to the most flexible person in the class.

For the next three years I continued to live on an extreme diet while I completed teacher training in Oki-do yoga, a demanding Japanese style. Initially I consumed just fruit—two months of only watermelon, a month of mangos, a month of apricots—and then a more varied diet of fruit and salad. During the time of eating only fruit I reached an incredible level of flexibility, vitality and health. I could do 108 backflips in five and a half minutes. My body and mind had never felt better— the only drawback was that I had no friends. My lifestyle was so extreme that I couldn't relate to people anymore on a level where I could go to their house and share a meal.

After the course finished and I received my first teaching certificate, one of my best early teachers, Eve Gryzbowski, announced that an instructor was needed for a class in Newtown. No one raised a hand. She addressed me directly: 'Simon, do you have a reason why you can't take it?' I couldn't think of a reason fast enough and before I knew it she 'volunteered' me for that class, which I still happily take today, twenty years on.

Up to that point in my life there had been two people whom I would call important teachers: one was my father, which I will explain later, the other was a Tibetan lama [teacher] whom I met when I was seventeen and who taught me some of the philosophy of yoga. I remember him telling me that we each have a special gift that we bring to the world. I said that at seventeen I doubted that I had any but he replied, 'Simon, your gift is empathy.' My Tibetan lama gave me so much information that I couldn't assimilate it for years and even ten, fifteen years later I would suddenly understand something and then realise that this lama had told me that many years before.

Soon I met two more people who affected my life as significant teachers. In 1985 I learnt there was to be a workshop given by Shandor Remete. I had heard a lot about Shandor, how he liked to shock students and how powerful a teacher he was. I enrolled and turned up full of anticipation. As I entered the room I saw a man with his legs behind his head, his body glowing in perspiration and I was impressed. 'This must be him!' I thought. Then a tall, broad man walked in wearing a suave Armani suit and dark glasses and I suddenly realised that this was Shandor; the man on the mat was one of Shandor's students.

During the first session Shandor had us do one pose per breath. Coming from a background of aerobics and with my love of dance, I thought this was the best class I had ever done and afterwards I vowed to drive to Melbourne where he usually taught to study with him whenever possible. The next day we did the second session of the workshop and this time he made us do two hours of forward bends holding each pose for five or ten minutes and then finishing with *kurmasana* [legs over the shoulders, chest to the floor]. He had to manoeuvre me into this last pose and, after the ten minutes were up, prise me out of it too. After that class my legs were so stiff I couldn't walk properly for two weeks. But after the stiffness dissipated, I could bend forward easily; in that two-hour class he changed my hamstrings for good. More than my hamstrings, he changed my approach to practice. He taught me how to enkindle the drive that was within me to explore yoga. Of all the yoga teachers I have encountered Shandor would be the best I have ever known, but even more than that he is someone who inspires me to this day. He regularly gives workshops at our school, and when he is in Sydney I have the privilege of still practising with my mentor and dear friend.

The other person who over the years has become one of my best teachers is Bianca Machliss. After a year of spending time together, we started teaching and travelling to India and in 1990 established Yoga Synergy, which we have developed as a style of yoga and a business since. Over the years, while travelling around India, Bianca and I met more teachers who showed us many extreme and esoteric practices. We studied *ashtanga vinyasa* with an amazing old American yogi, Cliff Barber, who has long white hair and a chest-length beard, and who has walked barefoot for the last thirty years. In Pune we came across pole yoga [*mallakhamb*] and practised with the All Indian National *Mallakhamb* champions in the Maharasthra Mandal. These champions, who were between six and twenty-six years old, would confidently perform handstands and backbends on top of a wooden pole three metres high and no wider in diameter than an orange. This taught us a basic principle of the way we teach—practise with a balance between flexibility and strength, engaging muscles that you may not need to use to achieve the pose but that make it safer for the body.

One of our teachers, Professor Bhim, who won the 'All India Gold Medal in Yoga Competition' in 1973–74, even showed us feats such as slowing his heartbeat, lying on a bed of nails without drawing blood, tearing metal sheets in two with his bare hands and inflating a football bladder with his nostril. He could do all this because he had mastered the breath. And this is what we learnt: the most esoteric teachings always required the breath to be held in or out for a long period of time. How to breathe properly is a focal point of the way we teach Synergy-style yoga.

# THE POWER OF THE BREATH

When I was six years old my father, George Borg-Olivier, taught me how to swim underwater. He grew up in Malta. He didn't have much money when he was young, so he taught himself to dive to earn a living. Because the proper diving equipment was too expensive, he and two of his friends worked out how to hold their breath for long enough to skin dive into wrecked ships and stay there four or five minutes to retrieve objects and then return safely to the surface. Once he made the newspaper headlines because a school bus veered off a cliff and the driver was trapped deep under the water. My father happened to be there and dived into what was a freezing winter sea and was able to prise the door open and free the driver—all because he had taught himself how to hold his breath. He later taught me how to do this by taking slightly deeper than normal breaths and by gripping my chest and abdomen in such a way that I could retain the in-breath for longer. He also taught me the signs to watch for that indicate the breath has been held for long enough and any longer would be dangerous. These instructions were the beginnings of what I would later come to know as *pranayama*—specifically *kapalabhati*, *bastrika* and *antara kumbhaka* [inhale retention].

When I was eight years old we left Malta and migrated via England to Australia. On the ship I met a Rhodesian Olympic athlete called Basil Brown who gave me instructions on how to do the same exercises that my father taught me but by holding my breath out. He also taught me how to perform some yoga breath techniques, such as *uddiyana bandha* [controlled expansion of the chest muscles which draws the abdomen inward], *nauli* [isolating the rectus abdominis], *lauliki* [rolling the abdomen from side to side] and *bahya kumbhaka* [exhale retention].

What my father and Basil had taught me would help save my life a decade later. When I was in my teenage years I had a 'junior scientist accident' where I inadvertently mixed a bunch of chemicals that caused a bright green flash, flames and an explosion of chlorine gas. Horrified, I gasped and inhaled a cloud of what was equivalent to mustard gas. The gas caused lesions in my lungs and blisters along the lining, and I coughed so much I burst a lung and ended up with a pneumothorax. The doctors thought I was going to die. I was like a human beanbag, with air pockets from my thigh to my neck and down my arms, and as a result I developed asthma.

I discovered that the only thing that would ease the extreme wheezing was if I listened to my body. To alleviate asthma all I had to do was comfortably hold my breath out or in for as long as possible and then not panic when I resumed breathing. To confirm this, the asthma came back when I was doing a lot of Iyengar yoga in Pune, which did not emphasise breath retentions presumably on the grounds of safety, and when I was doing *ashtanga vinyasa* yoga, which tended to emphasise increased breathing and hyperventilation, presumably to help increase abdominal and chest strength and help increase flexibility by alkalising the blood.

When I resumed the breath retentions my body was profoundly affected, especially the spine. A full exhalation is related to *mula bandha,* and learning how to grip the lower abdominal muscles while taking a full inhalation is related to *uddiyana bandha* and learning how to expand the chest. This enabled me to lengthen my upper back and release my stiff neck. Although it is important to fully inhale and fully exhale,

I learnt that if I took full breaths too often in a practice I felt destabilised and spaced out due to constriction of the arteries to the brain. Excessive pressures in the body generated during certain breathing practices, especially during breath retention, are potentially very dangerous, which is why B.K.S. Iyengar and K. Pattabhi Jois wisely caution against the premature teaching of *pranayama*.

Learning to retain the breath sounds straightforward enough but there is a catch. Holding the breath in or out causes an increase in the body's carbon dioxide and carbonic acid [the acid formed when $CO_2$ is dissolved in the blood]. The body's physiology can only tolerate large amounts of acid if the body's pH is more alkaline, and an alkaline system is best generated if you minimise your intake of acid-forming foods. When I began eliminating acid-forming foods, like grains, processed foods and high protein foods, I did my best yoga. Conversely, the only way to sustain this sort of diet is to also engage in a *pranayama* practice, which leads to a net reduction in the amount of air one breathes throughout the day. I am vegan and live on raw fruits, salads and occasionally steamed vegetables. I haven't eaten bread or rice or legumes in years, and hardly ever any nuts. I know other people who have tried to eat like this have ended up extremely spaced out, emotionally labile or suffering adverse allergic reactions, because they don't practise correct *pranayama*.

An underlying principle of Synergy-style yoga is the harnessing of energy, or *prana*. The ability to move *prana* around the body at will is an important aspect of *asana* practice and the correct use of *mudras* and *bandhas* can bring energy and blood to any organ in the body and can rid them of toxins or poisons that have accumulated. Breath control [or *pranayama*] is also used in most of the unique yoga exercises known as *kriyas* and *mudras*: *kriyas* are 'cleansing processes' that literally purify the body inside and out; *mudras* are special gestures, postures and muscle-control exercises that regulate the flow of energy in the body. Most *kriyas* and *mudras* require the use of *bandhas*. *Bandhas* can be thought of as muscle locks or energy guides. On a physical level a *bandha* is a co-activation of opposing muscles of a 'joint complex'.

The breath is essential to managing and guiding *prana* around the body in a safe way. *Prana* is simply energy. There are physical forms of energy—like sugar from food which travels in your blood, and adenosisne triphosphate (ATP), which is the main energy source of each cell—and there are energetic forms of energy, like the heat that your blood gives off. Then there is energy from light. I believe we are able to harness the energy of the sun in our body and this is why in India you see so many naked *sadhus* and *babas* [yogis and holy men]. To cover themselves in clothes would be to lose their inherent abilities to absorb *prana* from the sun. Many molecules that we know to be part of the photosynthetic complex of plants are present in the body. The basic structure of haem—as in haemoglobin in blood—is almost identical to the structure of chlorophyll. I find it hard to imagine that something so structurally similar can have no functional similarity as well. This is one of the reasons I generally practise outdoors and with minimal clothing.

Often in yoga classes people are told: 'Breathe!' The paradox is that if you take less breath the brain and the cells of the body actually get more oxygen (provided you periodically empty your lungs completely). This contributes to the saying that the yogi counts their life not in years but by the number of heartbeats and breaths they take.

When you hear people doing deep, fast breathing they are blowing off carbon dioxide before it has a chance to accumulate. The accumulation of carbon dioxide is a necessary stimulus that tells the blood vessels of the brain and lungs to open. If you breathe too much and diminish your $CO_2$ levels then the blood vessels shrink instead. Like the blood vessels to the brain, the bronchial tubes expand with the presence of carbon dioxide. Hence someone who hyperventilates (over-breathes) can end up with restricted oxygen levels and the possibility of having an asthma attack. Conversely, someone who hypoventilates (under-breathes) can get more oxygen into the lungs and therefore into the body's cells. This is of course an over-simplification as hyperventilation can be useful at times for the yogi for increasing flexibility, improving bowel movements and for preparing to hold the breath, but it is hypoventilation that leads the yogi to the more profound meditative states that characterise the essence of yoga. Hence, we place emphasis in our teaching on minimal breathing, taking long slow breaths and increased breath retention for those who are able.

## SYNTHESISING DIFFERENT STYLES

I had been practising yoga for many years when I began to get a niggling feeling that there was a link missing. From the very first yoga class I attended in 1983 through the fourteen times I studied in India until the mid-nineties I found that certain parts of my body were not being addressed in a way that was helping. In some cases my knees, lower back and neck were getting worse. I had been working with my own intense practice for some time when, through carelessness and overzealousness,

I injured myself. Worse, I heard of other yoga teachers who had things manifest in their bodies and this upset me.

A lot of people talk about injuries resulting from their yoga practice as if they are to be expected, but I never considered injury inevitable. Bianca and I went back to university as mature age students to study physiotherapy and health sciences, which ultimately taught us how to learn *about* the body. All of a sudden I knew how I could develop flexibility and strength where previously I had none, and how I could fix and heal longstanding injuries in my knees and my neck.

Our study of exercise physiology taught us to understand nerve reflexes and nerve tensioning (or stretching). The use of nerve reflexes in a yoga practice enables you to switch a muscle on when you want to use it, to turn it off when you need to relax it, and also how to increase strength and flexibility. The positions that I found best tension the nerves also stretch acupuncture meridians and closely resemble martial arts movements and classical *mudras* and gestures that you see in very old texts and in paintings on the walls of temples in India. There is a universal truth to the body, which is why you see many similar movements performed the world-round.

One of the most striking revelations from our study was that it wasn't what poses you did, but how you did them, and what you did before and after them, that made the biggest differences. Understanding of poses cannot simply be gained by copying an image. One must know whether to be pushing two parts of the body together in a pose or to be pulling them apart—or trying to keep them both passive. Each way has very different affects on the body.

A lot of classical yoga sequences are not functional for western bodies. These sequences assume lotus is relatively easy because Indians mostly sit cross-legged on the floor. They assume that deep squats like *utkatasana* and *malasana* are easy for everyone because most Indians squat to go to the toilet. And they assume the neck is already strong enough for inversions because most Indians carry loads on their head. Much of this is not true for westerners. If you change these assumptions and presuppose that you are starting out with a western body, then you need to address these differences between lifestyles and bodies with a warm-up of sorts. As Bianca and I have gradually refined our Synergy-style we find we are getting the best results from our students. It is not quite what we learnt from any one teacher or system but it is a synthesis of the knowledge we have gained from classical Hatha yoga and western medical science.

I learnt tremendous amounts from Mr Iyengar about how to work with *bandhas* throughout the body. On a scientific level a *bandha* is a simultaneous tensing of opposing muscles around a 'joint complex' and this is a central theme of the way we teach yoga. Through Mr Iyengar's intricate understanding of the symmetry of a pose, and the minutely detailed instruction he gives in order to reach it, he is creating *bandhas*, although he doesn't actually call them that. These are what make his postures effective in stabilising the main joints of the body and in directing flow of energy. In *Light on Yoga*, Iyengar refers to the three main *bandhas*, but the very use of the word 'main' in this context suggests there are more than just those three—*uddiyana*, *mula* and *jalandhara*—that yoga practitioners are most familiar with. This is what I have also found—*bandhas* exist throughout the body in each of the main joint complexes. It took me many years to understand Iyengar's methodology but finally I have determined how to elicit responses throughout the body that will have similar potent affects. I don't profess to teaching in the Iyengar style (in the cold and drafty halls where I began teaching it didn't suit students to continuously stop their practice and fetch props) and it is my opinion that only one person teaches Iyengar-style and that is Mr Iyengar; however, I have enormous respect for him.

Similarly, I don't teach the *ashtanga vinyasa* method of K. Pattabhi Jois, but through studying with him on a number of occasions I gained an appreciation for working with the breath in postures. I also began to appreciate the power and the potency of practising several set sequences. The reality is that most people in the world will only ever practise the primary *ashtanga vinyasa* series, and not all of it at that. Maybe three to five per cent of practitioners will reach the second series. And fewer still will go to the third series and beyond. However the people I know who really derive benefits from practising *ashtanga vinyasa* are the ones who practise three or four or even five sequences. By changing the series from day to day, their bodies are able to progress without repeating inevitable small errors that can lead to injury. To vary one's yoga practice in this way is important because there is good evidence to suggest that if you continually repeat the same practice then you will get good at the bits you are good at but you may actually get worse at what you are not inherently good at. Further weakening of an inherently vulnerable part of the body is less likely to happen if you vary your practice a bit from day to day.

My understanding from speaking to T.K.V. Desikachar—whose father, Professor T. Krishnamacharya was K. Pattabhi Jois's teacher—was that he initially taught the *ashtanga vinyasa* sequences to young Brahmin boys from their teenage years to no later than about twenty-five. Middle-aged people who have never done exercise in their life may not be the best people to learn *ashtanga vinyasa*. In any respect the principle is what stuck with me: to learn a set sequence of postures is useful and the basic format of the *ashtanga vinyasa* sequence is a helpful template.

Synergy-style yoga includes teaching five set series that can be practised sequentially from day to day, but for the purposes of teaching we instruct each series over a nine-week period so that a student can properly learn each series before moving on to the next. There are easier and harder versions of each series, as well as a range of degrees of difficulty within each pose. Therefore, as long as a person is able to walk up the stairs, sit down on the floor and stand up again and bear weight on one leg, then all five series are attainable. I can give instructions for an advanced pose so that an experienced student and a beginner student can both do the pose in a way that is safe and appropriate for their body.

This concept of working with the individual who is in front of you I learnt from Krishnamacharya, through his books and through class interaction with his son, Desikachar. If you are teaching a bunch of young kids you can give a lot more in both posture and speed than you would give an elderly sick person. Krishnamacharya was perhaps the yogi who has most influenced the way we practise yoga in the west: his students included B.K.S. Iyengar, Jois and his own son, Desikachar. Although I never met Krishnamacharya, I have really enjoyed meeting Desikachar on several occasions and I have felt connected to him. Desikachar is a very wise, warm and loving man and he has a real heart—which is probably why his book is called *Heart of Yoga*. We have a photograph of his father in our school. He is sitting in *mulabandhasana*, his abdomen drawn up in *uddiyana bandha*. This picture inspires me so much because of the calmness, wisdom and energy it seems to emanate.

The other place I find inspiration that is calm and wise and abundant in energy is in nature. In India I would often go to forest dance parties with friends and dance all night, sometimes on our hands with our legs waving in the air, and when the music reached an ecstatic climax we would flick our legs overhead into a backflip. Although it doesn't sound like yoga, it was through free-form dancing like this in nature that I really started to learn about meditation through movement. It is so invigorating to dance for sixteen hours non-stop. Just before dawn I would go deeper into the forest and do an hour's inverted yoga practice by myself, and that would give me the energy to resume dancing until after sunrise and sometimes for the rest of the day. This changed my perception of yoga into a means of cultivating energy.

It was during this time, in the late eighties, of travelling to India and practising yoga for six or seven hours a day, dancing at night and fasting a lot, that my perception of life began to change. I began to experience altered states of consciousness, as if I had left my body and was happily astral travelling. I enjoyed these sensations very much and tried to do it often. However, once when I was unwell and I tried to leave my body I found that I could not. It was as if I were trying to leave my house before first putting things in order and I appreciated that I needed to make those connections between body, mind and soul. I realised that I was trying to escape the body when really I am alive to be in the body, and my perspective on life changed radically. I suddenly felt this deep reverence for life that I can only describe as love, but which I feel is directly linked to what Patanjali calls *Ishvara pranidhana*. Because it was in this state of immense love that I felt a strong connection between my self and a higher Self, my spirit and body, my body and the earth, the earth and everyone on it. That feeling, a connection with all of life that emanates from the heart, became my focus. This I see as being at the core of yoga.

Can you take others there? I think B.K.S. Iyengar said it best when he said that you cannot teach someone how to meditate. What you can do is take them to a place where the conditions are right and they can practise, but they must learn to do it themselves. Similarly, perhaps, you cannot teach someone how to be 'spiritual'. It has to come to you and from within you. It helps to put yourself in the right environment and I think that yoga is the perfect environment. Yoga took a basic inclination I had for empathy and harnessed it. It helped me in all aspects of my life but especially in how I relate to other people: my wife, my friends, my students. It is one thing to make the connection between the body, the mind and the soul, but in a way that is the easy part. The real yoga is the yoga of relationships; the art is being able to embrace all those around you.

By practising you learn that yoga is a model for life. If you can approach life the same way you approach your yoga practice—by becoming more accepting, more tolerant to sensations that you might call pain—then your attitude, moods and responses to life and the people in your life will also change. It was my own ill-health and injury that first led me to yoga and now I try to help others on a physical level by relieving their back pain or neck pain. I know that in the greater scheme of life I only scratch the surface with what I do, but the practice is such that, of its own accord, it goes from the simple level of helping a physical problem, to addressing a physiological problem, to changing deeper mental and emotional issues. These are the stepping stones that lead to happiness on an individual level, that proceed to happiness on a group level and that eventually enable the whole world to become a better place.

# GLOSSARY

**Advaita Vedanta:** the philosophy of Oneness, belief in a singular universal essence that pervades all existence. (*Literally:* non-duality)

**Aghora:** an extreme path of Tantric yoga practice. Focuses on the underbelly of life in order to perceive the oneness of all existence. (*Literally:* non-terrifying)

**Aghori:** one who practises and is accomplished at Aghora

**ahamkhara:** the ego that defines our personality and limits our perception of our true nature, the Self. (*Literally:* I-maker)

**ahimsa:** non-harming; non-violence; the first of the five *yamas*

**antara kumbhaka:** breath retention used in *pranayama* after an inhale

**Arjuna:** the Pandava prince whose discussion with his charioteer, Lord Krishna, constitutes the *Bhagavad Gita*

**asana:** physical posture; the third limb of yoga as codified by Patanjali in the *Yoga Sutras*. (*Literally:* seat)

**ashtanga:** the eight limbs of classical yoga codified by Patanjali in the *Yoga Sutras*. The eight limbs are: *yama* (five moral observances), *niyama* (five self restraints), *asana* (postures), *pranayama* (breath practices), *pratyahara* (withdrawal of the senses), *dharana* (concentration), *dhyana* (one-pointed focus) and *samadhi* (ecstatic absorption). These combine as a spiritual practice to lead ultimately to *moksha* (release from ignorance of one's true nature) and *kaivalya* (liberation)

**ashtanga vinyasa:** a dynamic style of Hatha yoga taught by Sri K. Pattabhi Jois at the Ashtanga Yoga Research Institute, Mysore, India

**atman:** the Self

**avalokshena:** 'to look down upon'

**Avalokiteshvara:** from Tibetan Buddhism, the buddha that looks down upon humanity with compassion. (*Also:* Chenrezig)

**avidya:** ignorance; the primary cause of suffering; neglecting awareness of one's constant and true nature, the Self, and of the universal nature of existence, Oneness.

**Ayurveda:** traditional system of Indian medicine. (*Literally:* 'the science of life')

**baddha konasana:** name of a physical pose, seated with knees bent and feet together

**bandha:** contraction of muscles to intentionally conduct and direct energy in the body. (*Literally:* 'bond'; 'lock')

**Bhagavad Gita:** profound philosophical instruction from Lord Krishna to Arjuna about right duty in life. (*Literally:* 'Song of the Lord') The ancient text first appeared as a passage within one of India's great epic poems, the *Mahabharata*. (*Also:* the *Gita*)

**Bhakti yoga:** emphasis in practice is on devotion to a god or goddess (*deva/devi*) as a means to understand the nature of all existence

**Brahma:** first god of the Hindu trinity who governs worldly creation. (*See also*: Vishnu and Shiva)

**chakra:** major energy junctures in the body. (*Literally:* wheel of energy)

**Chaya Samyukta:** Shadow yoga

**chela:** disciple

**citta:** consciousness

**citta nadi:** mindstream

**deva:** gods; divine entities

**devi:** goddesses; divine entities

**dharma:** spiritual law; code of spiritual path

**guru:** spiritual teacher. (*Literally:* light in the dark)

**Hanuman:** mythological monkey chief who rescued Sita from her captors and returned her to her beloved, Rama, the hero of the epic poem, the *Ramayana*

**Hatha yoga:** yoga practice where emphasis is on physical posture, cleansing practices, breath work and meditation

**Hatha Yoga Pradipika:** a text on Hatha yoga, the physical disciplines and spiritual goals, written in the fourteenth century by sage Swatmarana

**Iyengar yoga:** the method of Hatha yoga that emphasises exactness of alignment in *asana*, originating from B.K.S. Iyengar and the Iyengar family at Ramamani Iyengar Yoga Institute, Pune, India

**Ishvara pranidhana:** faith in and surrender to the existence of a greater all-pervasive, all-knowing energy. (*Also:* the Lord; Spirit; God)

**jalandhara bandha:** one of three main locks used in Hatha yoga formed by contracting muscles in the chin/throat region

**janu sirsasana:** name of physical pose, seated forward bend. (*Literally*: head to knee pose)

**Jyotisha:** Vedic astrology

**Kalachakra:** a form of Tibetan Buddhism meditation practice. (*Literally*: cycle of time)

**kapalabhati:** a form of *pranayama* practice that cleanses the energetic body

**karma:** the consequence of any action with which one self-identified while performing

**Karma yoga:** yoga practice where emphasis is on dedicating one's actions and service to the benefit of others and to the transcendence of *ahamkhara*. (*Also:* selfless action, awareness in action)

**kirtan:** group-singing of Sanskrit mantras and hymns

**koshas:** the five layers that are intermeshed to comprise the individual: *annamayakosha* (the food cover, gross physical form); *pranamayakosha* (the life-force body, subtle form); *manomayakosha* (the mental body, subtle form); *vinjamayakosha* (the wisdom body, subtle form); and *anandamayakosha* (the bliss body, casual form)

**Krishna:** celebrated hero of Indian mythology, in particular in the *Bhagavad Gita*

**Krishnamurti:** Indian philosopher and author

**Kriya yoga:** emphasis on meditation to transcend personality–self to higher Self; style of yoga taught by the Self-Realization Fellowship founded by Paramahansa Yogananda, author of *Autobiography of a Yogi*

**kula devata:** family deity

**kundalini kriyas:** advanced practice combining bodily replace-ment and gestures to reach higher states of consciousness

**lauliki:** churning of isolated abdominal muscles to cleanse digestive organs. (*See also:* nauli)

**Mahasamadhi:** conscious decision to leave the body. Euphemism for death of a great person

**Mahavakya:** Great truth

**marmashastra:** study of energy points (*marma*) on the body

**mala:** a garland of prayer beads

**maya:** illusory nature of existence in the world

**mayurasana:** name of a physical pose, balancing on the elbows; the peacock

**moksha:** ultimate freedom from suffering when one ceases to self-identify with the ego-mind and instead resides in the Self

**mouna:** internal silence

**mudra:** a psychic expression made as a physical gesture that alters the flow of energy in the body

**mula bandha:** one of three main bodily locks used in Hatha yoga, formed by contracting the perineum, to redirect the body's flow of energy

**muladhara chakra:** the base chakra

**nadi:** subtle energy pathway in the body

**nadi shodhana:** a form of *pranayama* that cleanses and bal-ances the energy pathways

**Natarajasana:** name of a physical pose. Nataraja is Lord of the Dance, a name of Shiva who dances in continuous destruc-tion and recreation of the universe

**nauli:** isolating the abdominal muscles. (*See also:* lauliki)

**nivritti eye:** inward focused awareness

**niyama:** five behavioural principles by which yogis abide: *shaucha* (cleanliness), *santosha* (contentment), *tapas* (fervour, burning effort), *svadhyaya* (study of the Self), *Ishvara pranidhana* (faith in God, surrender to the Lord); the second limb of classical yoga

**padangustha danurasana:** name of physical pose; lying on stomach and forming a 'bow' by holding on to one's toes overhead

**padma:** lotus (*padmasana:* lotus position for meditation)

**parampara:** lineage of teachings passed from guru to disciple over generations

**Patanjali:** Indian sage who lived around 150 BC and who first codified yoga in the *Yoga Sutras*

**pinda:** embryo, foetus

**pitta:** Ayurvedic constitution that is dominated by the elements fire and water

**prana:** life-giving energy

**pranayama:** rhythmic breathing techniques to focus the mind and enhance one's prana; the fourth limb of classical yoga

**pratyahara:** inward turning of the five senses away from stimuli in the external sensory world towards the subtleties of the internal world; the fifth limb of classical yoga

**Radha:** consort of Krishna

**rishi:** one who has mastered yoga and has perceived the truth of existence. (*Literally:* seer)

**rnanubandhanas:** the bondage of karmic debt

**sadhana:** spiritual practice

**samadhi:** ecstatic absorption in the object of one's meditation

**samakonasana:** name of physical pose; the side splits

**samskara:** residual traits of the personality from past actions or lifetimes

**sannyasin:** one who has renounced the material world for the spiritual world. (*Equivalent:* monk)

**Sanskrit:** ancient language of India

**sattva:** harmony and balance; one of three cosmic forces. (*Also: rajas,* excessive activity; *tamas,* underactivity)

**sattvic:** harmonising cosmic force

**Shakti:** feminine form of the Divine; Tantric belief that Shakti is the creative energy behind the dynamic Cosmos

**shala:** room

**shaucha:** purity, cleanliness

**shishya:** disciple

**Shiva:** the third god of the Hindu trinity who governs destruction. (*See also:* Brahma; Vishnu)

**Sita:** wife of Rama, hero of the epic Ramayana

**sloka:** Sanskrit verse

**smashan:** cremation grounds

**supta virasana:** name of a pose; lying back between bent knees

**sthana:** alternative name for the practice of physical postures. (*Literally:* bodily placements)

**summa iru:** leitmotif meaning 'simply be'

**svadhyaya:** study of the texts; self-study

**svadisthana chakra:** the second lowest chakra, seat of creation in the body

**swami:** one who has gained mastery over themself. (*See also:* sannyasin)

**Tantric yoga:** a main branch of yoga based on the Tantras (sacred texts). The right-hand path of Tantra follows conservative spiritual practices, while the left-hand path follows unconventional spiritual practices to the same end

**tamasic:** cosmic force of underactivity; inertia

**trikonasana:** name of pose, standing triangle

**uddiyana bandha:** one of three main physical locks used in Hatha yoga formed by contracting the muscles of the abdomen and diaphragm

**Umma:** maternal name to denote the creative force behind all existence. (*Literally:* Mother; *also* Ma; Great Goddess)

**upavishta konasana:** name of a physical pose; seated forward-bend with legs wide

**vasana:** desires; tendencies that cause one to act out patterns of behaviour

**vayu:** wind; currents of energy in the body

**Vedanta:** philosophy of the Vedas (*See also:* Advaita Vedanta)

**Vedic:** pertaining to the Vedas, ancient philosophical hymns composed over 5000 years ago

**viparita chakrasana:** name of physical pose, backflips

**Vishnu:** one of the gods in the Hindu trinity who governs preservation. (*See also*: Brahma; Shiva)

**yama:** the first of the eight limbs of classical yoga. Five moral observances by which a yogi abides: *ahimsa* (non-harming), *satya* (truthfulness), *asteya* (non-covetousness), *brahmacharya* (moral living) and *aparigraha* (non-grasping)

**yantra:** sacred geometric symbol

**yoga nidra:** a practice of deep relaxation. (*Literally:* psychic sleep)

**yoga:** a way to transcend personality and connect with one's eternal, constant nature. From Sanskrit root 'yuj', to bind, to yoke

**Yoga Sutras:** composed by the sage Patanjali, an ancient text of 196 aphorisms in four chapters that codify the path of classical yoga. The key yogic text

**yogasana:** *see* asana

# BIBLIOGRAPHY

Simon Borg-Olivier and Bianca Machliss, *Applied Anatomy and Physiology to Hatha Yoga*, Yoga Synergy, Sydney, 1995

Baba Ram Dass, *Be Here Now*, Crown Publishing Group, New York, 1976

W. Y. Evans-Wertz, *Tibetan Yoga and Secret Doctrines*, Oxford University Press, London, 1935

Donna Farhi, *The Breathing Book*, Henry Holt, New York, 1996

——*Yoga Mind, Body & Spirit: A Return to Wholeness*, Henry Holt, New York, 2000

——*Bringing Yoga to Life: The Everyday Practice of Enlightened Living*, Harper San Francisco, 2003

B.K.S. Iyengar, *Light on Yoga*, George Allen & Unwin, London, 1966

Maggi Lidchi, *Earthman*, Victor Gollancz, London, 1967

Swami Muktananda Saraswati, *Nawa Yogini Tantra*, Bihar School of Yoga, Monghyr, Bihar, India, 1977

Antoine de St-Exupcry, *Wind, Sand and Stars*, Heinemann, London, 1954

Swami Prabhavananda and Christopher Isherwood (trans.), *How to Know God: The Yoga Aphorisms of Patanjali*, Vedanta Press, California, 1953

Swami Satyananda Saraswati, *Meditations from the Tantras*, Bihar School of Yoga, Monghyr, Bihar, India, 1974

Robert E. Svoboda, *Aghora: At the Left Hand of God*, Brotherhood of Life, Inc., Albuquerque, New Mexico, 1997

——*Aghora II: Kundalini*, Brotherhood of Life, Inc., Albuquerque, New Mexico, 1993

——*Aghora III: The Law of Karma*, 1998, Brotherhood of Life, Inc. & Sadhana Publications, Albuquerque, New Mexico

Swatmarana, *Hatha Yoga Pradipika*, trans. Pancham, Sinh, SSP, New Delhi, 1979

Selvarajan Yesudian and Elisabeth Haich, *Yoga and Health*, George Allen & Unwin, London, 1953

Paramahansa Yogananda, *Autobiography of a Yogi*, Self-Realization Fellowship, California, 1946

# RECOMMENDED FURTHER READING

Paul Brunton, *A Search in Secret India*, Samuel Weiser, New York, 1977

T.K.V. Desikachar, *The Heart of Yoga: Developing a Personal Practice*, Inner Traditions, Rochester, Vermont, 1995

T.K.V. Desikachar and R.H. Cravens, *Health, Healing & Beyond: Yoga & the Living Tradition of Krishnamacharya*, Aperture Foundation, New York, 1998

T.K.V. Desikachar with Martyn Neal, *What are we Seeking?*, Krishnamacharya Yoga Mandriam, Channai, India, 2001

Eknath Easwaran (trans.), *The Upanishads*, Nilgiri Press, California, 1987

Georg Feurstein, *The Yoga-Sutra of Patanjali*, Inner Traditions, Rochester, Vermont, 1990

——*The Philosophy of Classical Yoga*, Inner Traditions, Rochester, Vermont, 1996

——*The Shambhala Encyclopedia of Yoga*, Shambhala, Boston, 2000

Georg Feurstein and Jeanine Miller, *The Essence of Yoga*, Inner Traditions, Rochester, Vermont, 1998

David Goodman (ed.), *Be As You Are: The Teachings of Sri Ramana Maharishi*, Arkana, London, 1985

B.K.S. Iyengar, *Light on Paranyama*, George Allen & Unwin, London, 1981

——*The Tree of Yoga*, Thorsons, London, 1988

——*Light on the Yoga Sutras of Pantanjali*, Thorsons, London, 1993

Geeta S. Iyengar, *Yoga: A Gem for Women*, Timeless Books, India, 1990

K. Pattabhi Jois, *Yoga Mala*, North Point Press, New York, 1999

Howard Murphet, *Sai Baba: Man of Miracles*, Muller, London, 1971

Ann Myren and Dorothy Madison (eds), *Living at the Source: Yoga Teachings of Swami Vivekananda*, Shambhala, Boston, 1993

Swami Niranjananda Saraswati, *Prana Pranayama Prana Vidya*, Bihar School of Yoga, Bihar, India, 1994

Swami Satyananda Saraswati, *Asana, Pranayama, Mudra, Bandha*, Bihar School of Yoga, Bihar, India, 1969

——*Kundalini Tantra*, Bihar School of Yoga, Bihar, India, 1984

Mukunda Stiles, *Yoga Sutras of Patanjali*, Weiser Books, Boston, 2002

Barbara Stoler Miller, *Yoga: Discipline of Freedom [The Yoga Sutra Attributed to Patanjali]*, Bantam Books, New York, 1998

Robert E. Svoboda, *The Hidden Secret of Ayurveda*, The Ayurvedic Press, Albuquerque, New Mexico, 1980

# WEBSITES

*actionyoga.com* The Action School of Yoga, Melbourne and schedule for Glenn Ceresoli workshops worldwide

*ayri.com* official site of ashtanga vinyasa yoga as taught by Sri K. Pattabhi Jois at the Ashtanga Yoga Research Institute, Mysore

*bksiyengar.com* the official website of Iyengar Yoga as taught by B.K.S. Iyengar at the Ramamani Iyengar Yoga Memorial Institute

*dhamma.org* official website for Vipassana meditation as taught by S.N. Goenka

*donnafarhi.co.nz* Donna Farhi workshop and teacher training schedule worldwide

*drsvoboda.com* Robert E. Svoboda's teaching schedule

*kataragama.org* the official website for the Pada yatra to the sacred temple in Kataragama, Sri Lanka

*satyananda.net* the official website for the Satyananda organisation, including a catalogue of publications and audio material

*shadowyoga.com* Shandor Remete's worldwide workshop schedule

*yogamoves.com.au* Eileen Hall's schedule and Ashtanga Yoga Moves, Sydney

*yogasynergy.com.au* Simon Borg-Olivier's schedule and Yoga Synergy, Sydney

*yrec.org* Georg Feurstein's excellent yoga resource

# PHOTO CAPTIONS
# AND CREDITS

# ACKNOWLEDGEMENTS

Reverence and thanks to: Muktanand Meannjin and Kundan, Donna Farhi, Glenn Ceresoli, Shandor Remete, Simon Borg-Olivier, Eileen Hall, Rose Baudin and Robert Svoboda for sharing their time, their stories and themselves. Special thanks to Muktanand who died before the book was completed—thank you for the trust and inspiration. To Annette Barlow, Colette Vella and everyone at Allen & Unwin who applied their skill and talent to this book to help make it manifest! To Mum, Rebecca Zipser, Alistair Bisset and Anna Du Chesne for insightful feedback and willingness to help transcribe! To Rick and Deb for constant support and guidance in bringing yoga into everyday life. To Nick, Anouk, my family, for the love and nurturing. Om shanti. Om.